Patient Advocacy

by Nichole Davis, DHA, MPH, BCPA

for dummies®
A Wiley Brand

Patient Advocacy For Dummies®

Published by: **John Wiley & Sons, Inc.,** 111 River Street, Hoboken, NJ 07030-5774, www.wiley.com

Published simultaneously in Canada

For general information on our other products and services, please contact our Customer Care Department within the U.S. at 877-762-2974, outside the U.S. at 317-572-3993, or fax 317-572-4002. For technical support, please visit https://hub.wiley.com/community/support/dummies.

Wiley publishes in a variety of print and electronic formats and by print-on-demand. Some material included with standard print versions of this book may not be included in e-books or in print-on-demand. If this book refers to media that is not included in the version you purchased, you may download this material at http://booksupport.wiley.com. For more information about Wiley products, visit www.wiley.com.

Library of Congress Control Number: 2025934654

ISBN 978-1-394-28108-4 (pbk); ISBN 978-1-394-28110-7 (ebk);
ISBN 978-1-394-28109-1 (ebk)

SKY10100994_032525

Contents at a Glance

Table of Contents

Introduction

Hello and welcome! Think of this book at your GPS navigation through the world of patient advocacy. Wanting to be a confident and informed consumer of the healthcare system as a patient is one thing, but being one is another. In this rapidly evolving healthcare landscape, now — more than ever — it's necessary to empower yourself with the effective advocacy strategies and techniques to keep you and your loved ones from being overwhelmed, lost, unheard, and potentially even unsafe on your journey.

This book bridges the gaps between imagining the healthcare journey you want and being on track to achieving it. Being a patient — or supporting one — comes with a lot of questions and emotions, and that's why you need an easy reference guide with actionable steps.

About This Book

I know you're busy, so I've organized this book in the easy-access way the *For Dummies* series is known for. You may choose to read the book from cover to cover, or you may read any section or chapter as it calls to you. Whether you're interested in revamping your entire dynamic with your clinical providers or in refining your current approach, this book contains clear explanations, simplified concepts, and actionable exercises to get started.

No matter where you are in your healthcare journey — whether navigating a new or existing illness, challenging a diagnosis, seeking better answers, or just wanting to be more prepared and in control of your healthcare journey, this book is written with you in mind to help you find your power as a patient and find your voice in every conversation regarding your care.

Foolish Assumptions

I know you're no dummy! But the world of healthcare and patient advocacy is complicated and vast, so I know you'll appreciate starting with the basics. You don't need a medical degree or any prior knowledge to benefit from this book. In fact, this book is the perfect first step in becoming a patient advocate, whether it's for yourself or for your loved ones, and I invite you to continue to explore further as you read and want to learn more about any of the topics covered here.

If you do have a medical background and want to understand your role as a patient advocate more deeply, this book will also serve you well. For you, I provide detail and a fair amount of depth across the spectrum, but always in a clear and direct manner.

Icons Used in This Book

Throughout the book, you'll notice little pictures in the margins. These icons point you to information that you may not want to forget or, in some cases, you may decide to skip over.

TIP

These tips point you toward helpful information that can make your journey as an advocate a little smoother.

REMEMBER

When I point to information for you to remember, that means I think it's worthwhile for you to pause and make a mental note of the information; it can help you down the road in your understanding.

WARNING

Please take note of all warnings. This icon indicates pitfalls and hazards you might run across in the healthcare world.

FIND ONLINE

This icon alerts you to additional information you can find online that will help you on your healthcare journey.

Beyond the Book

In addition to the book content, you can find valuable free material online. I provide you with a Cheat Sheet that addresses questions that may be first and foremost in your mind. Check out this book's online Cheat Sheet by searching `www.dummies.com` for **Patient Advocacy for Dummies Cheat Sheet.**

Where to Go from Here

Patient Advocacy For Dummies is both an introduction and a beginner's reference. It's serves you whether you're advocating for yourself or for a loved one. You can read the chapters one after the other and follow along, or you can dip into the book here and there, reading up on the subjects that currently interest you.

If you're a newcomer to the role of a patient advocate, I recommend that you spend some time with the table of contents and leaf through the book to get a general sense of how I have structured and approached the material. You probably want to begin your reading with the first three chapters, which give you a picture of the current landscape.

If you want a refresher, or need a topic-specific insight, you can also use this book as a reliable guide in answering your questions. Perusing the table of contents is a good starting point for you as well. You may find yourself gravitating to later chapters that zero in on specific issues, such as advocating for your child's healthcare needs or dealing with chronic and long-term conditions. And of course, the index is always useful to locate specific information on any topic of interest.

Whether you're completely new or already somewhat familiar with the role of patient advocacy, you're in the right place. This book guides you through the briars so you can confidently advocate for yourself or for your loved ones, no matter what the circumstances dictate.

1 Getting Started with Patient Advocacy

IN THIS PART . . .

Understanding what a patient advocate does, how they help, and why you need one

Deciphering medical terminology, understanding medical records, and addressing errors

Unraveling the complexities of Medicare and healthcare coverage

Learning what informed consent is and how it protects your rights

IN THIS CHAPTER

- Participating in your own care
- Understanding what a patient advocate does
- Differentiating between types of patient advocates

Chapter 1 Finding Your Compass Through the Healthcare Maze

Welcome to the sometimes frustrating journey of healthcare advocacy. Whether you're advocating for yourself or for a loved one, this process can be difficult, but this book can help you along the journey. This book is for patients, their caregivers, including friends, family, and others — anyone who helps someone else manage and navigate the healthcare system. Whether you are reading this book to advocate for your own health or you are an active participant in helping someone else manage this experience, this book can help.

The U.S. healthcare system is complicated and multifaceted. It's sometimes nearly impossible to figure out what's best for your care and how that corresponds with what you can afford. In order to be an effective advocate during the healthcare journey, you need to be educated and understand the diagnoses, treatment plans, side-effects, costs, and more. The goal of this book is to help you become the best advocate you can — for your own care as well as for your loved ones'.

Participating in Your Own Care

If you're like most patients, the idea of "consuming" the healthcare system probably sounds a bit odd. Healthcare doesn't feel like something you consume, right? You get sick, go to a doctor, they tell you what to do, you follow along, and you hope to get better. That's the classic model of paternalistic medicine, which is the way the process worked for years. But things have shifted, and healthcare professionals now lean toward *participatory care*. Here's the thing: Not all patients have caught on to this change, and that disconnect can make all the difference in your healthcare experience.

Being a *participant* in your care isn't about pushing your doctor around or being demanding — it's about understanding that you have a right to safe, accurate, and effective care. Whether you're paying with insurance or out-of-pocket, you're investing in a service, and like any consumer, you have the right to expect a standard of quality.

However, to participate fully, you to need continually educate yourself about your condition and possible treatments; keep your records, medications, and treatments organized; and have the time and peace of mind to ask the right questions. If that sounds daunting, you are not alone (see Figure 1-1). It might be time to seek out an advocate who can help.

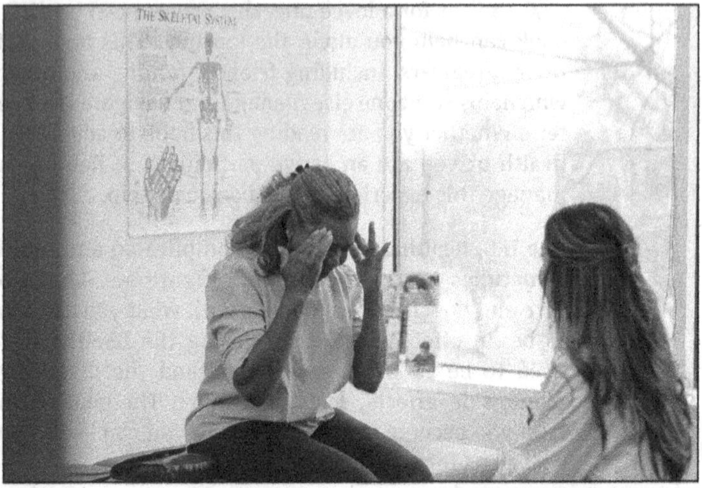

SDI Productions/Getty Images

FIGURE 1-1: If you find trying to understand and advocate for your own healthcare daunting and stressful, finding a professional advocate is a great idea.

Understanding Patient Advocacy

Patient advocacy, at its core, is a simple concept: it's about helping a patient achieve the outcomes they want and need in their care. Anyone — family, friends, healthcare professionals, and patients themselves — can step into the role of a patient advocate. But while anyone *can* advocate, the quality and impact of advocacy varies greatly depending on who's providing it and how it's done. Just like anything else, effective advocacy requires understanding, commitment, and a genuine focus on the patient's best interests.

Patient advocacy as a patient

Patient advocacy, when you're doing it for yourself — what I call *patient self-advocacy* — is all about standing up for your own best interests regarding your healthcare. To do this properly, you need to:

- Stay informed about your health
- Ask questions about your care plans
- Understand how each part of your healthcare journey support your well-being

You may not realize it, but you're probably already advocating for yourself in many ways. For example, when you tell your clinician that you're having stomach pain and you'd like to know why and seek treatment, you're taking an active role in seeking the care you need.

Patient advocacy as a support partner

When you advocate for a patient as a support partner — whether you're their spouse, friend, family member, or someone else who you care about — you're there to help ensure they receive the care they need and deserve.

Your role is about actively supporting them: asking questions they might miss (with their permission, of course), keeping them accountable to their care, and helping them feel confident and understood as they navigate their healthcare journey. It's about being their voice when needed, but also respecting their wishes, making sure that the care they receive aligns with their values and preferences.

Patient advocacy as a provider

Many healthcare providers — doctors, nurses, nurse practitioners, and physician assistants — advocate for their patients by going beyond simply performing their clinical duties. They make sure their patients don't slip through the cracks in complex healthcare processes.

For instance, a provider may recognize that a patient's symptoms call for a specialist and actively push for that referral, ensuring the patient gets the targeted care they need. They might also step in to help navigate insurance challenges, advocating for coverage when claims are denied or costs become a barrier to necessary care.

Providers bring not only their expertise but also a commitment to their patients' best interests, often working behind the scenes to secure the resources and attention their patients require.

Differentiating Types of Patient Advocates

The term *patient advocate* is used widely across different healthcare roles, often creating some confusion. In some companies, customer service representatives are called patient advocates, while hospitals might give this title to financial liaisons, care managers, or other staff. While these roles do involve advocacy for patients, it's useful to understand that the nature of their advocacy can vary based on their responsibilities, their employer, and their relationship to your care.

Institutional/hospital patient advocates

You may have heard about someone called a patient advocate who works for the hospital. Sometimes these professionals are called case managers, care coordinators, or navigators, among other names. These are individuals employed by the hospital to help patients connect their care between providers, answer questions, and improve the patient's experience. The work that these professionals do is very meaningful, especially for patients admitted to the hospital who have many moving parts to their care.

It's important to recognize, however, that these individuals are employed by and work for the hospital. That means their assistance only stretches so far. When a patient is discharged from the hospital, or transferred to another facility, this hospital employee may no longer provide any hands-on assistance.

They're there to help patients have a better healthcare experience, but they ultimately still work for the hospital. They can be a resource for you as an advocate, but you can't rely on them to be a full patient advocate as you (or your loved one) navigate different stages of care.

TIP

You may also hear the term patient advocate used in other spaces too, such as for the representative who helps you when you call your insurance company, or the individual who works at a hospital ombudsman office to help you file a complaint. This term is used in many areas to mean anyone who might help a patient with healthcare issues.

Private patient advocates

Private or independent patient advocates provide patient advocacy services independent of a healthcare system and are often contracted or hired directly by the patient or their family to provide personalized assistance, regardless of where the patient is receiving care.

Many private and independent patient advocates provide different types of services depending on the needs of their clients and the advocate's area of expertise. If they don't provide the service that you're looking for, ask if they have any recommendations of advocates that do. The work that these professionals do is extremely collaborative and that doesn't just mean with the healthcare teams their clients work with — they may also collaborate with other patient advocates and know of different contacts to help you with a specific need.

Some private patient advocates carry industry certifications to show that they have demonstrated expertise and specialize knowledge in different areas of the healthcare navigation process, along with the bonus of showing how committed they are to the provision of high-quality advocacy.

- A private patient advocate who has achieved the credential Board Certified Patient Advocate or BCPA, has met specific competencies established by the Patient Advocate Certification Board (PACB) that speaks to their knowledge of the healthcare system, their grasp on patient rights, the role of a patient advocate on a healthcare team with a patient, and more.

- Some advocates hold the Certified Case Manager or CCM certification that is awarded to them by the Commission for Case Manager Certification (CCCM) proving that they have mastered case management skills, like care coordination.
- Advocates that hold the certification of Certified Senior Advisor or CSA, have a passion for working with older and aging patients as clients and have demonstrated their understanding of the unique needs, both clinically and otherwise, that specifically affect seniors in the healthcare system.

Do your research and learn as much as you can about the private patient advocate you are considering working with. One size does not fit all and you want to make sure you have a connection with, and work well with, the professional you add to your healthcare team.

Most advocates require that you complete a consultation call for meeting with them so that they can fully understand your needs, your expectations, your currency, and what your goals are. Some advocates don't charge for consultations, while others do.

Friends and family members as advocates

When a friend or loved one gets sick, it's common for their loved ones, such as family members and friends, to step in and support their journey to wellness. Having someone by your side who is familiar and can support you as you navigate the healthcare system is very important, and patients often find solace in members of their support network.

Family and friends do a wonderful job supporting their loved ones, to the extent that they're able. However, the healthcare system is confusing, even if your loved one or friend has experience with it. As you involve your loved ones in your care, manage everyone's expectations about what that support looks like. As well-meaning as they may be, you might need more help ensuring your healthcare journey moves along smoothly.

Navigating the Healthcare System

You likely realize by this point that the U.S. healthcare system is quite flawed. However, there's also a great deal of people who are committed to making it work. The aim of this book is not only to educate you but also to empower you with the realization that you don't have to always take what you're given or navigate your journey alone.

Remember, you have options, you have power, and your perspective is important and relevant to your care. This book is now one of your resources to navigate that journey.

IN THIS CHAPTER

» **Learning important medical terms and abbreviations**

» **Getting help deciphering all the mumbo-jumbo**

» **Finding and reporting errors in your medical records**

» **Using health management tools**

Chapter 2
Decoding Medical Terminology and Records

Healthcare can feel like it's packed with confusing terms — some words might make sense if you sound them out, while others feel like a foreign language. But understanding basic medical terminology isn't just a "nice-to-have" — it's essential for being actively involved in your care. Medical professionals rely on this language to communicate about your treatment, and having a handle on key terms can make a big difference in how informed and confident you feel.

The good news is, you don't need a medical degree to get a grasp on the basics. By learning how to decode complex terms, you can more easily read and understand your medical records, spot any potential errors, and communicate clearly with your healthcare team.

Getting a handle on your health data — things like lab results, imaging, treatment plans, and more — gives you a clearer view of how your health is evolving over time. This awareness doesn't just make you more informed; it empowers you to actively participate in your care. When you're familiar with the key terms in your records and can understand how your data tells a story, you're better prepared to make informed decisions alongside your healthcare providers.

This chapter introduces you to essential medical terms and gives you tips on navigating healthcare jargon, so you don't feel like you're watching a foreign TV show without subtitles. Let's dive in!

Deciphering Medical Acronyms, Abbreviations, and Terms

By now, you've probably noticed: Not only do healthcare professionals use complex words with Greek and Latin roots, but they're also big on abbreviations and acronyms — especially in charting and notes. While it wouldn't be practical (or necessary) to memorize every abbreviation, learning some commonly used ones can help you feel more in control when reviewing your medical information.

Terms and abbreviations you're likely to see time and again include the following:

- **Acute:** Sudden or severe onset condition
- **Benign:** Not harmful, non-cancerous
- **BP:** Blood pressure
- **CBC:** Complete blood count, a common blood test
- **Chronic:** Long-term or ongoing condition
- **CT:** Computed tomograpy, a type of image scan, i.e. a CT scan
- **Dx:** Diagnosis
- **ECG or EKG:** Electrocardiogram
- **FX:** Fracture, broken bone
- **HPI:** History of present illness
- **HR:** Heart rate
- **Hx:** History
- **IV:** Intravenous

- **Malignant:** Cancerous
- **MRI:** Magnetic Resonance Imaging
- **Myocardial infarction:** A fancy word for a heart attack
- **OTC:** Over-the-counter
- **PCP:** Primary care provider, or physician
- **PMHX:** Past medical history
- **PRN:** As needed; can be seen in conversations about medication, like taking Tylenol PRN, or as needed
- **Pt:** Patient
- **Px:** Prognosis
- **Rx:** Prescription
- **Sepsis:** Extreme immune reaction to infection
- **Thrombosis:** Blood clot in a blood vessel
- **UTI:** Urinary tract infection

Taking a few minutes to familiarize yourself with these can help you follow conversations more comfortably.

FIND ONLINE

This isn't an exhaustive list, and resources like the Mayo Clinic's Glossary of Terms (`www.mayo.edu`) and WebMD's Medical Abbreviation Finder (`www.webmd.com`) can be helpful references. Figure 2-1 shows the dashboard of the Mayo site, which houses a trove of reliable and up-to-date medical information.

If you come across an unfamiliar abbreviation in your records or on a doctor's note, don't hesitate to ask your provider to explain it, or look it up using one of these reliable resources. Having these tools handy can make it easier to stay informed and engaged in your healthcare journey.

TIP

Also, if certain terms keep coming up, it might not be a coincidence. It may be a signal that that word or abbreviation is important to providing context about your care. Use the resources mentioned earlier to get clear definitions — these terms can give you useful context in understanding your care!

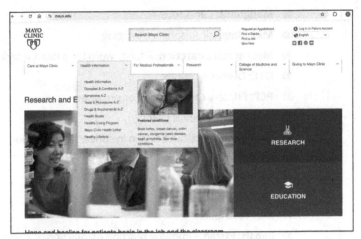

FIGURE 2-1: The Mayo Health Information site is a great source of medical information.

Latin and Greek prefixes and suffixes

Knowing some basic Greek and Latin root words can also go a long way into deciphering medical records and notes. Even just a few terms can help you:

- **Aqua-:** Pertaining to water
- **Asphyxia:** Choking or loss of consciousness due to oxygen deprivation
- **Carcin(o)-:** Related to or causing cancer
- **Cyto-:** Pertaining to a cell or cells
- **Derma-:** To do with the skin
- **Digit:** Either a finger or a toe
- **Encephal(o)-:** To do with the brain
- **Gastr(o)-:** Related to the stomach
- **Lact-:** Pertaining to milk
- **Men-:** A month or occurring monthly
- **Nephr(o)-:** Related to the kidneys
- **Onc(o)-:** To do with tumors or masses, often related to cancer
- **Ov-:** Pertaining to eggs (for example, ovulate)

- **Pulmon(o)-:** To do with the lungs
- **Stasis:** Causing the flow of a fluid, such as blood, to slow or stop
- **Viscous or viscosity:** Sticky or thick, thickness

By the same token, knowing these basic *prefixes* (found at the beginning of a word) and *suffixes* (found at the beginning of a word) can help:

- **A- or an-:** Lacking or without
- **Ab-:** Away from
- **-algia:** Indicates pain or a painful condition
- **Cardio-:** Related to the heart
- **Ecto- or exo-:** Outside of
- **-ectomy:** Removal through surgery
- **Hyper-:** Above, beyond or in excess
- **Hypo-:** Below, or not enough
- **-itis:** An inflammation
- **-mortem:** Relating to death
- **-plasty:** Repair through surgery
- **Post-:** After or behind
- **-rrhea:** A discharge or a flow
- **-somnia:** Related to sleep
- **Trans-:** Across or through
- **-trophic:** Relating to nutrition
- **Vas(o)-:** Relating to a vessel

Medical terms related to body systems

In addition to general medical terms and abbreviations for tests and procedures, you'll also come across key terms specific to different body systems, like the respiratory, gastrointestinal, endocrine, and cardiovascular systems. These terms often describe conditions or processes related to each system:

- HTN stands for hypertension (high blood pressure), which is linked to the cardiovascular system.

- DM is short for diabetes mellitus, or diabetes, a chronic condition affecting the endocrine system.
- COPD represents chronic obstructive pulmonary disease, impacting the respiratory system.
- CHF stands for congestive heart failure.

If you're managing a particular condition or working with a specialist, like a cardiologist, it's helpful to familiarize yourself with terms commonly used for that body system. Doing a quick search on medical terms specific to your condition or care area can give you a solid foundation.

TIP

You don't need to memorize or master each term's complex details, but having a general sense of what it means and what system it relates to can be useful across your healthcare interactions. For example, a term like HTN might show up in your past medical history, not only in your cardiologist's notes but also in records from other providers, giving you a clearer picture of your overall health history.

Navigating the terminology jungle

Understanding the common abbreviations and terms used in treating, assessing, and monitoring conditions like heart disease or cancer can empower you to better manage your care. However, no matter how much you learn or try to remember, it's likely that you'll come across terms that just don't ring a bell. That's okay and normal. Consider these practical tips for getting the answers to your questions:

- **Ask your healthcare team:** During your next appointment, ask for any patient education resources or handouts that explain key terms in simple language.
- **Use trusted disease-specific organizations:** Websites like the American Heart Association, National Multiple Sclerosis Society, or others related to your condition may offer resources to help you understand the terminology specific to your care.
- **Google it:** For quick explanations, look up unfamiliar terms, but make sure to cross-check with reliable sources.

- **Request clear explanations:** Don't hesitate to ask your care team to explain terms or abbreviations in plain English. For example, learning that "hypokalemia" means "low potassium" can make these terms easier to remember and understand in context. You can also write these terms down in your own healthcare notebook, or ask your care team to do it for you.

Assessing and Using Your Medical Records

To get your medical records, you can contact your health system and place a medical records request. You may be able to request your medical records electronically, so check with your health system for how to do so. You can request your entire record or just specific information. Be mindful that you may not get a copy of your medical records for a few weeks. There are costs associated with acquiring your records, so be sure to ask how much it will cost. Remember that information in your medical record is covered by the Health Insurance Portability and Accountability Act (HIPAA). Make sure you sign any necessary consent forms, especially if you are accessing medical records for someone else.

TIP

HIPAA (the U.S. Health Insurance Portability and Accountability Act passed in 1996) gives you the right to access your records and request changes to inaccurate or missing information. Ensuring your records are up-to-date isn't just a proactive step to better, safer healthcare — it's your right.

Your medical records are a key part of your healthcare story, serving as a comprehensive narrative of your well-being. They outline the basics of your medical history, giving you and your healthcare providers an overview of important details like past diagnoses, treatments you've had (or are currently undergoing), medications, family medical history, allergies, and more. Understanding your own medical history doesn't just help you keep track of what you've been through — it also allows you to see how your information is documented and shared across your care team.

Think of your medical history as a "resume" of your health. Just like a resume gives employers a snapshot of your education, work experience, skills, and other qualifications, your medical history gives healthcare providers a comprehensive summary of everything that's been happening with your care. From diagnoses that have been confirmed to treatments you're undergoing or conditions still being evaluated, your medical history paints the picture of where you've been and where you are now in your health journey.

WARNING

Accuracy in this "health resume" is essential. Just as an incorrect degree or omitted job experience on a job resume could impact your employment, missing or incorrect information in your medical records could affect your care. This is why it's important to access your records and review them regularly, ensuring they're complete, up-to-date, and correct. Keeping tabs on what's in your medical records means having an accurate, reliable picture of your health — a picture that could make all the difference in emergency situations or when coordinating long-term care.

Spotting errors: A beginner's guide to error resolution

Mistakes happen, even in your medical records. But why should you care if something's wrong? Well, errors in your records can lead to big issues. Imagine a serious allergy missing from your record or an incorrect medication dosage.

REMEMBER

Doctors rely on your records to make informed decisions that safeguard your well-being, so accuracy is vital.

Reviewing your records can feel overwhelming, especially if they seem like an endless scroll unraveling in front of you. Regular checks make it more manageable, so try to do a quick review after major events, like changes in your care plan, emergencies, surgeries, or other significant treatments. This helps you spot any new errors before they pile up over time. Also, two sets of eyes is always better.

Checking for and fixing errors

Try these tips when checking your records:

- » **Confirm your basic info:** Make sure your contact details, like name, phone number, and birth date, are correct.

Errors in these can lead to mix-ups, especially if you have a common name.

- **Check past diagnoses and medical history:** Be sure that listed diagnoses are accurate and not just "possible" or "under evaluation."
- **Update allergies and surgeries:** Ensure these are current and specific. For instance, if you had surgery on your right shoulder, it shouldn't show up as a left shoulder surgery.
- **Bring in a second pair of eyes:** Ask a trusted family member, patient advocate, or friend to help review. Another perspective can be valuable for catching mistakes.

If you find an error, here's what to do:

- **For smaller issues,** like a wrong phone number, contact your doctor's office for a quick fix.
- **For bigger errors,** like a misdiagnosis, submit a formal written request to correct it. You might need to provide documentation to back up the correction, so ask about the required information and timeline.

If you're hitting a wall, you have options:

- **Start by clarifying:** Contact the hospital to understand why the error hasn't been fixed; sometimes, they need additional information from you.
- **File a complaint if needed:** If errors persist, you can file a complaint with the state health department.
- **Add a statement of disagreement:** For unresolved issues, you can add a note in your record indicating you disagree with the information.

REMEMBER

Accurate medical records are the backbone of effective care. By ensuring there are no errors in your records and staying curious about the details, you can improve communication with your healthcare team, spot potential trends in your health, and bring meaningful questions to your appointments, making your voice an integral part of the decision-making process.

Familiarizing Yourself with Health Management Tools

Patient portals available through your health system can be valuable tools for managing your healthcare. These online platforms give you direct access to your provider's notes, let you view test results, and often include secure messaging so you can communicate directly with your providers.

Portals can also help you stay on top of important health information like symptom management and lab results. For instance, if you're monitoring glucose levels for diabetes, you can check trends in recent lab values and discuss them with your clinician through the portal.

TIP

If you aren't sure whether your healthcare provides uses a portal (they likely do) or how to access it, start by calling the main desk and asking. They can give you the website information and explain how to log in and set up an account. It's not much different than signing up for Amazon or any other website account.

In addition, consider using health apps to support your day-to-day management. Many apps let you track symptoms, set medication reminders, and even connect data with your healthcare providers, making it easier to update them on your progress. Some popular apps include MedisafeApp for medication reminders, Flo for menstrual health tracking, and MyFitnessPal and Apple Health for overall health management insights.

IN THIS CHAPTER

- » Understanding Medicare coverage
- » Explaining in-network vs. out-of-network
- » Finding the best prices on prescription drugs
- » Navigating coverage changes

Chapter 3
Unraveling the Knots of Health Insurance

Navigating healthcare is one thing — finding ways to afford it is another. Many individuals within the American healthcare system are covered by some form of health insurance. This may include private insurance obtained through employers or the marketplace, coverage provided by military service through the VA (veterans affairs department), or government programs like Medicare and Medicaid. But how does this complex system operate? Who shoulders the financial burden and to what extent? What happens if you're eligible for only one type of insurance? What if you have overlapping coverage or none at all?

This chapter guides you through the fundamentals of health insurance, illustrating its impact on both your healthcare journey and financial responsibilities. By the end of this chapter, you'll feel empowered and ready to engage in meaningful discussions about coverage, out-of-pocket expenses, and avenues to secure insurance. So buckle up — this is an important part of the journey!

Understanding the Differences Between Medicaid and Medicare

Two of the most popular healthcare coverages in the United States are Medicare and Medicaid. Although they are often mentioned together, they are different coverages with different roles.

- Medicare, for the most part, supports older adults, meaning people over 65 years old, as well as people with disabilities.
- Medicaid supports people who have lower incomes, disabilities, young children, and more.

Medicare requirements do not vary from state to state but Medicaid requirements do. It's possible for someone who has Medicare to also have Medicaid and vice versa because they are eligible for both coverages, such as an older adult who is in the low income bracket. In some instances Medicaid pays for services that Medicare does not pay.

The ABCs (and D) of Medicare Coverage

For many patients, health insurance is complex enough on its own, but Medicare adds an extra layer of complexity. Medicare is a federal health insurance program in the United States. People over the age of 65 or who have certain recognized disabilities are eligible to receive it. Medicare can be used to pay for healthcare expenses like trips to the hospital and many other healthcare services that other insurance companies will cover.

Medicare has unique rules governing what's covered, how it's covered, and for how long, and it interacts with other types of insurance in ways that are distinct from other payers.

Each part of Medicare covers different aspects of healthcare needs — one part focuses on inpatient hospital stays, another on outpatient care, like emergency department visits, and more. Understanding how these parts work together can help you navigate your coverage, anticipate what's covered during healthcare discussions, and gain more control over unexpected costs.

According to the U.S. Department of Health and Human Services, a person may be eligible for Medicare if they:

- Are aged 65 years or older
- Have a qualifying disability, such as a diagnosis of end-stage renal disease (ESRD), which is permanent kidney failure, or amyotrophic lateral sclerosis (ALS), also known as Lou Gehrig's disease

FIND ONLINE

For a deeper understanding of eligibility criteria and how they apply to your situation, check out resources from the U.S. Department of Health and Human Services (at hhs.gov), which offer detailed guidance on Medicare eligibility and enrollment.

Don't worry — you don't need to be a Medicare expert to start. This chapter provides a clear, straightforward overview of each part of Medicare to give you a strong foundation. You'll gain a better grasp of how Medicare works so you can use it effectively as a patient and understand its role in your care.

Basics of Medicare Part A

Medicare Part A primarily covers inpatient hospital stays, hospice care, some home health services, and care in skilled nursing facilities. When a patient is admitted to the hospital, Part A generally covers related services, including meals, nursing, and medications administered during your stay.

If you or your spouse worked and paid Medicare taxes for at least ten years, you may qualify for Part A without a monthly premium. For more details on eligibility, visit medicare.gov or consult your care team, as there might be additional eligibility criteria for those who don't meet the work history or age requirement but meet other requirements.

WARNING

Even if you qualify for premium-free Part A, there are still out-of-pocket costs like deductibles, co-pays, and co-insurance — terms you might associate with other insurance types. Medicare Part A covers a large portion of hospitalization costs, but the length of your hospital stay affects coverage levels. For example, Medicare may cover 100 percent of your costs for the first 60 days, but from day 61 onward, you may need to share the costs.

Deductibles also apply to Medicare Part A. The *deductible* is the amount you pay out-of-pocket before Medicare starts covering your care. Being eligible for Part A doesn't guarantee that you'll automatically have other parts of Medicare, like Part B, which covers outpatient services. Some people only have Part A, covering inpatient costs, while other expenses, like doctor's visits, remain uncovered by Medicare.

Make sure to familiarize yourself with the specific deductibles, co-pays, and the number of days covered under Medicare Part A for different services, such as hospital stays and skilled nursing facility care. This knowledge will help you plan for potential expenses and avoid surprises along the way.

FIND ONLINE

Don't assume you're automatically enrolled in Medicare Part A just because you've turned 65. You may need to actively apply through the Social Security Administration. This can be done at a Social Security office, over the phone, or on the `medicare.gov` site. Make a note a few months before you turn 65 to start the enrollment process, as you don't receive any reminders about your eligibility.

WARNING

Just because you stay overnight at the hospital doesn't necessarily mean you're considered "admitted." In some cases, patients stay overnight under "observation" status, which is typically an outpatient designation. This matters because observation stays are billed differently and typically fall under Medicare Part B or other insurance coverage for outpatient services. If you only have Medicare Part A and stay overnight under observation, you could face a hefty bill since Part A generally won't cover observation stays. Before you agree to stay overnight, ask your clinician to clarify if you're being admitted as an inpatient or staying for observation. This distinction has a big impact on how your hospital stay is billed.

Basics of Medicare Part B

Medicare Part B focuses on outpatient care and preventive health services, such as doctor's visits, emergency department care, mental health services, and medical equipment like wheelchairs or walkers. Part B also covers some preventive care, including annual wellness exams and screenings to detect health issues early. However, it doesn't include services like dental or vision care, most prescription drugs (except in special cases), or hearing aids. Many patients rely on additional insurance, such as Medicaid or a private plan, for these types of services.

Most people pay a monthly premium for Medicare Part B. While there's a standard premium, higher-income individuals may pay an increased amount, known as the Income-Related Monthly Adjustment Amount (IRMAA). Like Part A, Part B has a deductible that you must meet before coverage starts. After the deductible, Part B typically covers 80 percent of approved costs, with patients responsible for the remaining 20 percent — either themselves or on their behalf by using a another coverage to cover it.

FIND ONLINE

For up-to-date information on current premiums and deductibles, refer to `medicare.gov`.

TIP

Enrolling in Medicare Part B on time is crucial to avoid late enrollment penalties. These penalties are intended to prevent people from waiting to sign up for Medicare once they're sick and in need of coverage. You have a seven-month initial enrollment period that starts three months before your 65th birthday and ends three months after. Missing this window can result in a penalty, increasing your monthly premium for each year of delayed enrollment.

Timely enrollment not only spares you from ongoing penalties but also enables you to access Medicare coverage as soon as you're eligible. Keep in mind that these penalties don't go away; they can stick with you for as long as you have the coverage (which could literally be for the rest on your life *cue music for dramatic effect*). So, signing up on time can save you a significant amount in the long run!

Basics of Medicare Part C (Medicare Advantage)

You now know that Medicare Part A covers inpatient care, and Part B handles outpatient services — so what's Medicare Part C all about?

Medicare Part C, also known as *Medicare Advantage*, is like a bundled, all-in-one alternative to original Medicare (Parts A and B) and often includes Part D (prescription drug coverage). Medicare Advantage combines inpatient and outpatient coverage with prescription coverage into a single plan, making it a streamlined option for those looking to simplify their healthcare coverage. Some Advantage plans even include services the original Medicare doesn't cover, like dental and vision care.

REMEMBER

Medicare Advantage works a bit differently than original Medicare. It usually operates with network restrictions, similar to plans you may have heard of, like PPOs (Preferred Provider Organizations) or HMOs (Health Maintenance Organizations).

This means that your coverage might be limited to a specific network of doctors and facilities, although you may find lower out-of-pocket costs as a tradeoff. If you want more flexibility to choose your providers without network restrictions, original Medicare might be a better. For example, patients who travel frequently and want the freedom to visit any hospital that accepts Medicare may opt for original Medicare over Medicare Advantage plans.

Consider these tips for picking the best plan for you:

- **Evaluate your healthcare needs:** Think about the services you use now and what you may need in the future. For example, if you see a lot of specialists, make sure the Advantage plan you're considering includes those providers in-network. If you know that vision care is important to you, compare the specific benefits each Medicare Advantage plan offers to maximize benefits.
- **Make sure your current provider network is covered:** Use a checklist of your current clinicians and hospitals and see if they're covered under the Medicare Advantage plan you're considering. It can be disruptive to lose access to trusted providers, so double-check this in advance.
- **Compare costs and get real about your budget and cash flow:** Medicare Advantage plans vary in monthly premiums, deductibles, and out-of-pocket costs. Decide if you prefer lower monthly premiums with potentially higher out-of-pocket costs when care is needed or a higher premium with lower expenses down the line. Make sure to be honest about your financial situation — there's no benefit in selecting a plan that stretches you beyond your budget.
- **Use the Medicare Plan Finder tool:** Visit `medicare.gov` to use the Medicare Plan Finder tool (see Figure 3-1). This resource allows you to compare plans based on various factors that matter to you, such as coverage types and costs.

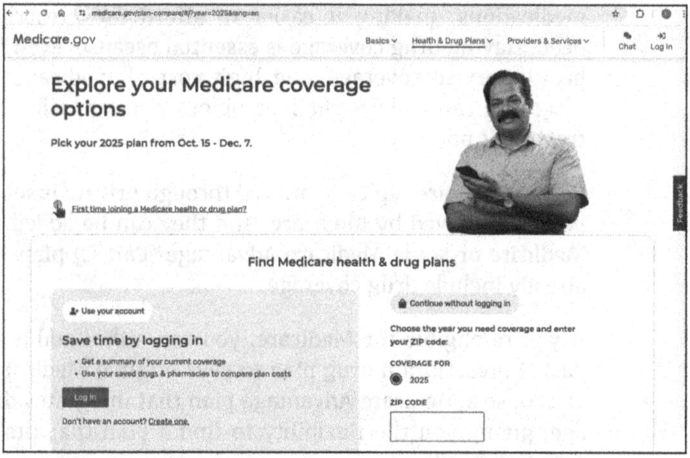

FIGURE 3-1: The Medicare Plan Finder tool helps you compare plans and find the one that benefits you most.

Ultimately, selecting the right Medicare plan is a personal decision. Consider your current and future healthcare needs to make an informed choice. Although Medicare Advantage could provide you flexibility and additional coverage that original Medicare may not, also take time to evaluate and work with your support team if it makes more sense to have original Medicare or to opt for an Advantage plan. The only right answer in this conversation is the option that is right for you.

TIP

You're not locked into one plan forever (unless you want to be)! As your healthcare needs evolve, so might your need for coverage. Make it a habit to review your Medicare plan each year to ensure it still meets your needs. If it doesn't, consider switching to a plan that's a better fit.

Except for certain special circumstances, the best time to make changes is during the annual *open enrollment period*, which is from October 15 to December 7 every year. This review process ensures that you're always getting the coverage that suits your current lifestyle and priorities.

Basics of Medicare Part D: Prescription drug coverage

One of the easiest parts of Medicare to remember is Part D — for *drug* coverage. Medicare Part D helps cover the cost of prescription medications, making it easier to afford the prescriptions you need. Having drug coverage is essential because, even if you have health service coverage, the high cost of medications without insurance can make it challenging or even impossible to follow a treatment plan.

Part D plans are typically offered through private insurance companies approved by Medicare, and they can be added to original Medicare or some Medicare Advantage (Part C) plans that don't already include drug coverage.

If you're eligible for Medicare, you can either add a standalone Part D prescription drug plan to your original Medicare coverage or choose a Medicare Advantage plan that integrates drug coverage, giving you the flexibility to find a plan that fits your prescription needs.

Formulary tiers and drug cost variation

Every part D plan has its own *formulary*, which is an offering of medications that are covered and organized into tiers. Make it a point to review the medications on your plan's formulary on a regular basis because sometimes they can change — a drug that may have been covered may not be covered in the future or an uncovered drug may now be covered.

Generally, there are four tiers:

- **Tier 1:** Includes generic drugs, generally offering the most affordable out-of-pocket costs.
- **Tier 2:** Incudes plan preferred brand-name drugs, requiring a moderate co-payment.
- **Tier 3:** Includes non-preferred brand-name drugs with a higher co-payment.
- **Tier 4 (and sometimes Tier 5):** Includes specialty drugs with the highest out-of-pocket cost.

Where your medication falls within these tiers can significantly affect your out-of-pocket costs. To save money, ask your clinician if you can start with a generic drug, or if a brand-name drug is necessary, pick one from the preferred tier. Remember, generics often perform just as well as their brand-name counterparts, although specific cases may necessitate a different approach.

WARNING

While generics work well for many people, some patients find that certain brand-name medications to be more effective for them. Discuss these options with your clinician to strike a balance between effectiveness and cost.

Verifying that the medication is necessary

Take the time to also ask your provider if the medication being prescribed is necessary. It may sound like a difficult thing to challenge, because why would your provider prescribe you a medication that is not necessary? Some medications may help provide comfort or address issues that are not critical, and you can ask your provider whether they feel like the medication is medically necessary for your condition. They can help you identify other alternatives to get the job done. You may want to have this conversation with your provider if you're faced with taking an expensive medication.

Medicare D has a prior authorization restriction called "step therapy," which requires you to try certain comparable drugs before covering a more expensive or non-preferred medication. This process helps manage costs but may require patience as you work through options to find what's best for you. As always, you can learn more about these drug plan rules at `medicare.gov`.

Understanding In-Network vs. Out-of-Network Coverage

Think of *in-network* and *out-of-network* coverage like having a loyalty card for a specific grocery store chain:

- **In-network (loyalty store):** Imagine you have a loyalty card for "For Dummies Foods." When you shop at any For Dummies Foods store (in-network), you get discounts and special deals and earn points because you're a loyalty member. Every time you shop there, you save more and enjoy the perks.
- **Out-of-network (non-loyalty store):** Now, if you go to a different grocery store that isn't part of the For Dummies Foods chain (out-of-network), your loyalty card doesn't work. You can still buy groceries, but there are no special deals, and you may end up paying higher prices because you're not a member.

With health insurance, *in-network* providers are like the "For Dummies Foods" stores — they have agreements with your insurance company to offer services at a lower cost. But if you go *out-of-network*, it's like shopping without your loyalty card at a non-affiliated store — you'll probably pay more and miss out on discounts or perks.

In-network providers and services have a pre-existing agreement with your insurance company to provide you services at a pre-negotiated rate that is often less expensive to you. Networks are created by insurance companies to help manage the cost of care and improve access to it to patients.

Common network types

You know those letters on the front of your insurance card, like HMO, PPO, or something similar? They actually mean something, even if most people don't know what that is right away. Here's a quick rundown of the most common types of networks:

- An **EPO** (Exclusive Provider Organization) gives members access to a limited set of providers without (usually) requiring referrals to see specialists.
- An **HMO** (Health Maintenance Organization) requires members to use in-network providers but usually allows exceptions in emergencies.
- A **PPO** (Preferred Provider Organization) offers flexibility by covering both in-network and out-of-network providers, although out-of-network services typically come with higher costs.

It's a good idea to stay informed on any changes to your insurance network — providers can move in and out based on contract renewals and other adjustments, which can impact your options for care.

Costly misconceptions about networks

Having insurance is great, but it doesn't guarantee cost-free access to any healthcare provider. It's important to understand your coverage limits to avoid unexpected expenses, especially when it comes to out-of-network providers who can charge substantial fees.

Emergency care and out-of-network coverage

The Emergency Medical Treatment and Labor Act (EMTALA) ensures you receive necessary emergency care, even at out-of-network hospitals. Keep in mind, though, that your insurance might not cover all costs incurred during out-of-network emergency department visits. An empowering tip is to identify nearby in-network emergency departments ahead of time.

TIP

Identify nearby in-network emergency departments in advance to avoid costly surprises during a crisis.

Proximity doesn't mean coverage

Remember, just because a healthcare facility is conveniently located near you doesn't mean it's in your network. While insurance companies are working to improve access and broaden their networks, there might still be gaps. By double-checking beforehand (see the section "Locating in-network providers," later in this chapter for how to do this), you can shield yourself from unexpected costs and ensure seamless access to affordable care.

Verify specialist and second opinion coverage

When you're referred to a specialist or seeking a second opinion, never assume that the provider is in-network. Always verify their coverage status under your plan by either calling your insurance company or checking your health plan's provider directory (also called Find a Doctor) online. It's a simple step that can significantly impact your healthcare budget and the quality of care you receive.

Double-check with your insurance provider

Reach out directly to your insurance provider to ensure providers and services are still in-network. Since networks can change annually, a provider covered last year might not be this year. Staying up-to-update on your coverage helps you make informed, cost-effective health decisions, empowering you to manage your healthcare confidently.

Locating in-network providers

Figuring out if a provider is in-network can feel like a guessing game, but thankfully there are tools to make it easier. Here are some reliable ways to keep your searches quick and accurate:

- **Use your insurance company's online directory:** Most insurers offer an online directory where you can search for in-network providers by location, specialty, or even specific names. It's a convenient way to access updated listings.
- **Download your insurance company's app, if available:** Many insurance companies now have apps that offer more than just basic info. These apps often feature tools to search for nearby in-network providers, view benefits, manage claims, and make payments. Some apps even use GPS to indicate local in-network providers on a map.
- **Call customer service for help:** Prefer a personal touch? Call the customer service line and ask a representative to help you verify if a particular provider is in-network. If you're searching in general, provide your ZIP code, and they can point you toward nearby options.

Several independent platforms now help patients find in-network providers, making it even easier. If you want a no-frills approach to quickly gathering most up-to-date info specific to your plan, your insurance provider's resources are a solid place to start.

Financial implications of in-network care

Using in-network providers and services can save you significant money, as out-of-network services often come with higher co-pays, co-insurance rates, or in some cases, may not be covered at all — leaving you responsible for the full bill. It's essential to recognize that healthcare delivery, your overall wellness, and financial planning are all interconnected. Take the time to learn which providers and hospital systems are part of your plan's network, which services are fully or partially covered, and any restrictions on where you can receive care.

WHAT IF YOU CAN'T AVOID OUT-OF-NETWORK COSTS?

TIP

Sometimes, despite your best efforts to stick with in-network providers, the unexpected happens. You might get food poisoning at a wedding across the country and end up in an out-of-network emergency department, or receive a call from your clinician during a road trip directing you to the nearest hospital — which isn't in your network. While you should make it a habit to use in-network providers, it's wise to budget for potential out-of-pocket costs associated with out-of-network care.

Integrate a contingency plan into your annual healthcare financial strategy to account for potential out-of-pocket costs linked with out-of-network care. Even though you don't expect to use it, take time to understand the additional co-pays, co-insurance, and out-of-pocket expenses that come with out-of-network services, and set aside a small amount each month for this purpose, if you can. This planning can help you handle the financial impact of an unexpected health emergency more smoothly if it ever arises.

If you already have an established care team, verify that each member is in-network to avoid unexpected expenses. Health insurance alone doesn't ensure protection from steep expenses; understanding what your plan covers, how much it covers, and under what circumstances can help you avoid financial strain. Viewing healthcare decisions holistically, inclusive of financial consideration, will better prepare you to minimize unpredicted medical expenses, decrease unnecessary out-of-pocket costs, and fully optimize your health insurance benefits.

Understanding VA Health Insurance: The Basics

Veterans Affairs (VA) health insurance is healthcare coverage specifically for veterans who meet certain service requirements, like having served active duty, among other criteria. Not only can the veteran who served be eligible for these benefits, but their spouse or other dependents may also qualify under specific conditions.

Eligibility and priority for VA insurance can depend on factors like service history, income level, disability rating, and more.

FIND ONLINE

Veterans can apply for VA insurance in person at a VA facility, online at `www.choose.va.gov`, by phone via 1-877-222-8387, or by mail by filling out the VA Form 10-10EZ, shown in Figure 3-2.

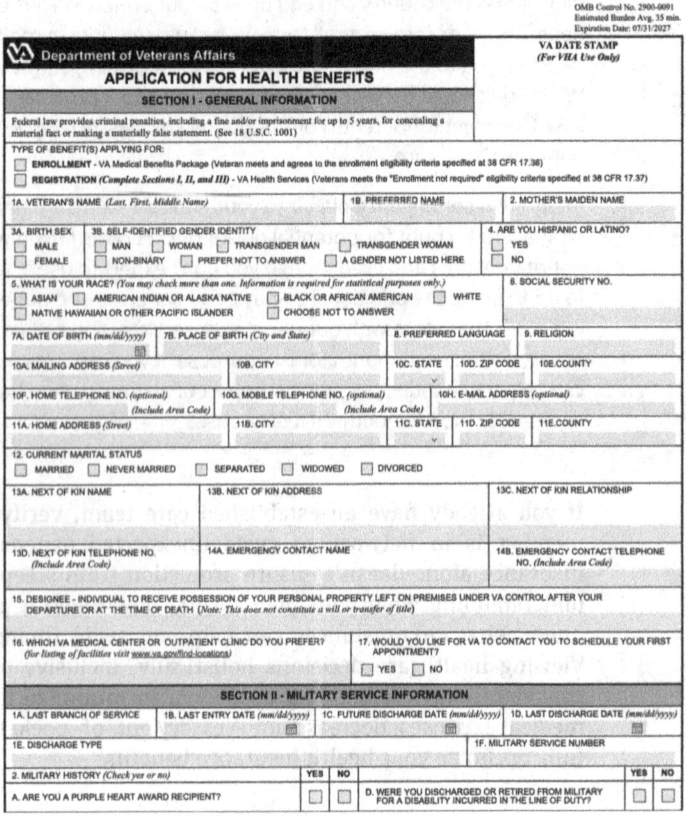

OMB Control No. 2900-0091
Estimated Burden Avg. 35 min.
Expiration Date: 07/31/2027

Department of Veterans Affairs

VA DATE STAMP
(For VHA Use Only)

APPLICATION FOR HEALTH BENEFITS

SECTION I - GENERAL INFORMATION

Federal law provides criminal penalties, including a fine and/or imprisonment for up to 5 years, for concealing a material fact or making a materially false statement. (See 18 U.S.C. 1001)

TYPE OF BENEFIT(S) APPLYING FOR:

☐ **ENROLLMENT** - VA Medical Benefits Package (Veteran meets and agrees to the enrollment eligibility criteria specified at 38 CFR 17.36)

☐ **REGISTRATION** *(Complete Sections I, II, and III)* - VA Health Services (Veterans meets the "Enrollment not required" eligibility criteria specified at 38 CFR 17.37)

1A. VETERAN'S NAME *(Last, First, Middle Name)* | 1B. PREFERRED NAME | 2. MOTHER'S MAIDEN NAME

3A. BIRTH SEX ☐ MALE ☐ FEMALE | 3B. SELF-IDENTIFIED GENDER IDENTITY ☐ MAN ☐ WOMAN ☐ TRANSGENDER MAN ☐ TRANSGENDER WOMAN ☐ NON-BINARY ☐ PREFER NOT TO ANSWER ☐ A GENDER NOT LISTED HERE | 4. ARE YOU HISPANIC OR LATINO? ☐ YES ☐ NO

5. WHAT IS YOUR RACE? *(You may check more than one. Information is required for statistical purposes only.)* ☐ ASIAN ☐ AMERICAN INDIAN OR ALASKA NATIVE ☐ BLACK OR AFRICAN AMERICAN ☐ WHITE ☐ NATIVE HAWAIIAN OR OTHER PACIFIC ISLANDER ☐ CHOOSE NOT TO ANSWER | 6. SOCIAL SECURITY NO.

7A. DATE OF BIRTH *(mm/dd/yyyy)* | 7B. PLACE OF BIRTH *(City and State)* | 8. PREFERRED LANGUAGE | 9. RELIGION

10A. MAILING ADDRESS *(Street)* | 10B. CITY | 10C. STATE | 10D. ZIP CODE | 10E.COUNTY

10F. HOME TELEPHONE NO. *(optional)* *(Include Area Code)* | 10G. MOBILE TELEPHONE NO. *(optional)* *(Include Area Code)* | 10H. E-MAIL ADDRESS *(optional)*

11A. HOME ADDRESS *(Street)* | 11B. CITY | 11C. STATE | 11D. ZIP CODE | 11E.COUNTY

12. CURRENT MARITAL STATUS ☐ MARRIED ☐ NEVER MARRIED ☐ SEPARATED ☐ WIDOWED ☐ DIVORCED

13A. NEXT OF KIN NAME | 13B. NEXT OF KIN ADDRESS | 13C. NEXT OF KIN RELATIONSHIP

13D. NEXT OF KIN TELEPHONE NO. *(Include Area Code)* | 14A. EMERGENCY CONTACT NAME | 14B. EMERGENCY CONTACT TELEPHONE NO. *(Include Area Code)*

15. DESIGNEE - INDIVIDUAL TO RECEIVE POSSESSION OF YOUR PERSONAL PROPERTY LEFT ON PREMISES UNDER VA CONTROL AFTER YOUR DEPARTURE OR AT THE TIME OF DEATH (*Note: This does not constitute a will or transfer of title*)

16. WHICH VA MEDICAL CENTER OR OUTPATIENT CLINIC DO YOU PREFER? *(for listing of facilities visit www.va.gov/find-locations)* | 17. WOULD YOU LIKE FOR VA TO CONTACT YOU TO SCHEDULE YOUR FIRST APPOINTMENT? ☐ YES ☐ NO

SECTION II - MILITARY SERVICE INFORMATION

1A. LAST BRANCH OF SERVICE | 1B. LAST ENTRY DATE *(mm/dd/yyyy)* | 1C. FUTURE DISCHARGE DATE *(mm/dd/yyyy)* | 1D. LAST DISCHARGE DATE *(mm/dd/yyyy)*

1E. DISCHARGE TYPE | 1F. MILITARY SERVICE NUMBER

2. MILITARY HISTORY *(Check yes or no)*	YES	NO		YES	NO
A. ARE YOU A PURPLE HEART AWARD RECIPIENT?	☐	☐	D. WERE YOU DISCHARGED OR RETIRED FROM MILITARY FOR A DISABILITY INCURRED IN THE LINE OF DUTY?	☐	☐

FIGURE 3-2: A quick look at the VA 10-10EZ form.

VA insurance covers a wide range of services, from preventive care and mental health support to prosthetics and specialized treatments, with care designed specifically for veterans and the unique needs they may have due to their service.

For many veterans, VA care is provided at no cost, but certain services may come with a co-payment. The cost structure often depends on whether a veteran has service-connected disabilities — many of these services are fully covered with little to no co-pay. Some veterans also qualify for free or reduced-cost medications, typically dispensed through VA pharmacies. Income levels and other factors can influence co-payment amounts and the availability of other financial support.

TIP

In cases where a VA facility isn't easily accessible or wait times are excessive, veterans may qualify for a Community Care program, allowing them to receive care from non-VA providers.

Veterans with VA insurance can also use other coverage they may have, like Medicare, Medicaid, or private insurance. The VA coordinates with those insurers to ensure accurate billing and to minimize costs for veterans.

For more details on VA health insurance benefits and how to apply, reach out to Veterans Affairs for specific guidance and information on available services.

Making Informed Decisions to Maximize Your Health Coverage

With all this information about the healthcare insurance world, you might be wondering why it's important to learn these details and apply them when making decisions about your care. The answer lies in the role that financial planning plays in accessing and paying for the resources and treatments you need. Think of it like house shopping — you wouldn't choose a dream home without considering your finances, credit score, and budget. While you might pick out a beautiful home, the reality of paying for it could be some serious rain on your parade.

Similarly, understanding your health coverage is key to making smart, informed choices about your care. In the United States, patients have financial obligations when accessing healthcare, whether they're paying out of pocket or through an insurance company. By learning about insurance, you empower yourself to make better choices, so that when it's time to "sign on the dotted line" for healthcare services, you're prepared and confident in your financial options.

TIP

For information about coverage gaps and for advice about solving billing errors, check out Chapter 12.

Researching and comparing plan options

Understanding your health plan is essential because not all plans are created equal. Each plan has unique features that impact your provider access, costs, and overall experience. Plus, as your healthcare needs evolve, the support you require may also change. Reviewing key details — like monthly premiums, deductibles, and out-of-pocket maximums — ensures that you get coverage that best aligns with your current situation. Consider these points:

- **Compare plans when you're considering a change:** When looking at a new plan, compare these elements to your existing plan so you're aware of any differences and changes to expect.
- **Think beyond monthly premiums:** While it's easy to focus on monthly costs, it's wise to consider total expenses over time. Sometimes paying a bit more each month can save you from larger bills later.
- **Ensure your care team is in-network:** This bears repeating. If you have a trusted care team, confirm they're in-network with your plan. This helps you avoid out-of-network costs or the need to find new providers.

Just like researching a treatment or medication, understanding your insurance plan can prevent future headaches. If navigating these details feels challenging, ask the finance department hospital or health system to provide you with patient education resources that can guide you on the right questions to ask and information to gather when picking a plan. For even more personalized support, consider working with an independent patient advocate who can help you make confident, informed decisions about your plan choice.

Taking a little time to evaluate these aspects can make all the difference in your healthcare experience, ensuring you have the right coverage without adding unnecessary financial stress.

Utilizing customer service and online resources

Customer service representatives at your insurance company can be helpful, especially when you need detailed, plan-specific information or a live person to talk through specific questions. Consider these points:

- **Get help:** When you call, you'll usually encounter an automated menu with options for claims, benefits, and more. If you're unsure where your issue fits, simply ask to speak with a representative who can direct you to the right area or provide a starting point for your inquiry.
- **Use online resources and tools:** Some insurance websites and third-party apps allow you to compare plans and estimate the costs of various medical services. While these tools may not offer official guidance, they can give you preliminary insights to discuss with your insurance provider, care team, or any support person helping you manage your coverage.

These resources are valuable for navigating the complexities of health insurance, enabling you to gather the information you need to make informed choices.

Using Price Comparison Platforms, Coupons, and Discounts

You've probably heard stories about this or even experience it in your own life — your medication may cost one amount at one pharmacy and be hundreds of dollars cheaper at another pharmacy. How do you manage this cost variability? How do you know the best prices and avoid filling your prescription wherever? Are there coupons? Can you even shop around for the best deals on procedures and medical services? Millions of patients have these questions and this section addresses them.

The benefits of "shopping around" for medications

Would you buy something at the first price you saw without checking for a better deal? Probably not! That same approach applies to buying medications, where prices can vary widely. Here are some practical ways to find the best prices and save on your prescriptions:

- **Check prices at different pharmacies:** Prices for the exact same medication can differ depending on the pharmacy or even your insurance plan. You can call the pharmacy directly or use the formulary lookup on your insurance company's website. You want information on the filling fee. You can also use price-comparison tools. By comparing prices, you might find savings that range from a few dollars to quite a lot, and that little bit of extra effort can make a big difference.
- **Explore discount programs:** Some medications come with discount programs that may actually beat what you'd pay with insurance — this is a great option if you have a high co-pay or if the medication isn't covered. Some of these programs are temporary, especially if a generic version hits the market, but it's always worth a look.
- **Try price comparison tools:** Apps and websites like RxSaver, GoodRx, and SingleCare are great resources for quickly checking medication prices across pharmacies. They often provide digital or printable coupons, which can mean instant savings.
- **Look into pharmacy membership programs:** Many pharmacies have membership programs that reward regular customers with discounts on prescriptions and other purchases. If you're filling prescriptions frequently, joining a membership program could save you even more.
- **Double-check discount eligibility:** If you're using a coupon or discount, be sure it's valid at your pharmacy. Some discounts have eligibility requirements, so it's a good idea to confirm with the pharmacy staff.
- **Chat with your pharmacist for extra savings:** Pharmacists and their staff often know about the latest discount programs, even ones that aren't widely advertised yet. Just ask; they may have a recommendation that could help you save.

- **Consider a longer prescription:** If it makes sense for your medication, ask your clinician, for example, about a 90-day prescription instead of a 30-day one. You might benefit from bulk pricing, and you'll cut down on the number of trips for refills.

Just a few extra minutes exploring these options can mean big savings on your medication, helping you keep more money in your pocket without sacrificing the care you need.

Getting the best deal on medical services

Shopping around for the best price on medical services, like CT scans or lab tests, is not just a cost-saving measure but also a way to actively engage in your healthcare decisions. Medical prices can vary widely, even within the same city, and understanding how to navigate this can make a big difference for your budget.

Here are some tips to help you make informed choices:

- **Understand the importance of the CPT code:** The CPT (Current Procedural Terminology) code is crucial as it precisely identifies the medical service or test you'll receive. This unique identifier allows you to accurately compare service fees, ensuring you're not left guessing in your healthcare decisions. Always ask your healthcare provider for the CPT code for any procedure you're planning to have and verify its accuracy. Without it, comparing prices can be like comparing apples to oranges.
- **Be bold about pricing transparency:** Contact the facilities where you might receive the test or procedure. Ask for a specific price estimate based on your insurance plan and the CPT code. Be direct and persistent if you need to be. Facilities should provide you with clear answers on how much you'll pay out of pocket, especially as healthcare transparency laws are increasing in many places.
- **Anticipate and inquire about additional fees and hidden costs:** Some facilities may not include all associated costs upfront. Ask if there are any additional fees — such as facility fees, interpretation fees (for imaging or labs), or any other charges beyond the primary procedure. This is especially

important for complex diagnostics like CT scans or MRIs, which may come with unanticipated charges.

- **Use comparison tools wisely:** Resources like Healthcare Bluebook, FAIR Health, and others can give you an idea of reasonable prices for various procedures in your area. However, be aware that these tools provide average estimates and may not reflect specific contract rates between providers and insurance companies. Use these tools as a starting point and verify actual prices with each facility directly.
- **Review your insurance benefits closely:** Some insurance plans have preferred facilities or labs that offer lower rates for specific tests. Verify if your insurer has a "preferred provider" network for diagnostic tests. Staying within this network can substantially reduce out-of-pocket expenses, and going outside it can mean higher out-of-pocket costs.
- **Check for real-time transparency information:** Many healthcare systems are now required by law to publish real-time pricing information online. Visit the websites of your preferred facilities to see if they offer price estimates for common procedures. While this information is becoming more accessible, it's still evolving, and not all hospitals or clinics offer detailed breakdowns yet.
- **Plan ahead when possible for elective and non-emergency procedures:** For non-emergency procedures, take the time to explore pricing and quality before scheduling. If you're having an elective test or an annual screening, this gives you time to do thorough research, which can lead to better savings and even a choice in quality care.

Using Health Savings Accounts (HSAs)

Health Savings Accounts (HSAs) can be a valuable tool for patients and families with high-deductible health plans (HDHPs), helping to save on out-of-pocket medical costs. An HSA offers tax advantages and allows you to save specifically for healthcare expenses if you're enrolled in an HDHP, which has higher deductibles but often lower monthly premiums than traditional insurance plans.

REMEMBER

One key benefit of an HSA is ownership — *you control the account*. This means the funds stay with you even if your employment changes or you stop working, offering you flexibility and financial support for medical costs. Eligible expenses for an HSA include deductibles, co-payments, and other health-related expenses, which you can verify on the IRS website. Just keep in mind that HSA funds are for healthcare only, so you can't use them on non-medical items, like dance lessons.

To learn more about HDHPs or HSAs, check with your insurance provider, HSA administrator at a trusted financial institution, or a financial advisor, tax professional, or patient advocate who specializes in insurance navigation. They can guide you on your options and how to make the most of your HSA benefits.

Navigating Changes in Coverage

Having health insurance now doesn't always mean it will stay that way or that you'll remain eligible. Life changes — like losing a job or moving from full-time to part-time — can impact your coverage. In such cases, you may qualify for COBRA, a federal program that temporarily allows you to keep your current insurance while transitioning to new coverage.

Other life events, like the loss of a spouse who provided insurance, might make you eligible for special provisions to change your health plan. Even if nothing changes for you, provider networks sometimes shift, and clinicians or facilities may stop accepting certain insurance plans. If this happens, you'll typically receive a notice via mail or your secure hospital messaging portal.

When you get this type of notice, it's essential to follow these steps:

1. **Confirm which aspects of your insurance are impacted (such as specific providers or types of care).**
2. **Evaluate how this affects your current care team.**
3. **Plan next steps with your provider.**

In some cases, you may need to discuss transitioning to a provider or system that remains in-network to ensure continuity of care. Having a plan can help you navigate these unexpected changes smoothly.

Getting the Care You Need Even When You Don't Have Insurance

If you find yourself needing care without health insurance, there are still options for managing costs and accessing support. While emergency medical services are your right, remember that the hospital can still bill you, even if you're uninsured. Patients in between coverage, who've recently lost coverage, or who don't have insurance, often worry about the quality of care they'll receive and the costs involved.

Here are some actions to consider:

- **Explore financial assistance programs:** Many health systems offer financial assistance programs, often available to patients with limited income. Even if you think you may not qualify, it's worth asking about the application process — you might be eligible for partial or full assistance.
- **Look into community health clinics and FQHCs:** Community health clinics and federally qualified health centers (FQHCs) offer free or low-cost health services. Many use a sliding scale fee structure, making them accessible to those without insurance.
- **Consider urgent care for non-emergency issues:** For non-emergent issues like sore throats or minor injuries, urgent care clinics offer a lower-cost alternative to the emergency department. Urgent care staff can also advise you if a more intensive emergency department visit is needed.
- **Try telehealth for low-acuity concerns:** Virtual care is often a cost-effective option, with some visits costing under $50. Telehealth can be helpful for minor issues and provide quick access to a healthcare provider. You can also remove the additional expense of getting to your appointment by logging on virtually.
- **Investigate special enrollment periods or Medicaid:** If you've lost coverage due to life changes, you may qualify for a special enrollment period, allowing you to apply for insurance outside the regular open enrollment window. If you meet income requirements, Medicaid may also be an option.

Exploring these options can help you maintain care and reduce financial stress during periods without insurance.

TIP

No matter your ability to pay, you have the right to be treated with respect and fairness, just like any other patient with insurance. If you feel dismissed, discriminated against, or disrespected due to not having health insurance, know that your patient rights are there to protect you.

In emergency situations, for instance, the Emergency Medical Treatment and Labor Act (EMTALA) ensures that emergency departments must provide care and cannot refuse treatment or transfer you simply because of an inability to pay. While EMTALA applies to emergencies only, you can still ask about payment options or financial assistance for non-emergency care.

Whether you're able to pay upfront or need to arrange assistance, no one has the right to treat you poorly. Your dignity as a patient should be respected in every setting.

IN THIS CHAPTER

» Understanding what informed consent is and how it protects your privacy

» Learning the essential components of an informed consent form

» Understanding the common challenges with the informed consent process

Chapter 4 Keeping the Power in Your Hands with Informed Consent

It's time to talk about and reframe *informed consent* — one of the most important tools you have to take charge of your healthcare decisions. You may think of the informed consent form as just a piece of paper you sign before you see your clinician, have surgery, or undergo a procedure or additional testing for a condition you have, but it is much more than that.

In this chapter, you learn why informed consent is pivotal to your patient self-advocacy efforts, the common components of an informed consent form, what questions to ask, and the resources you may need to ensure that you are confident about what you're signing.

What's the Big Deal? The Significance of Informed Consent

You may genuinely be asking yourself, "What is all this fuss over a consent form?" You have every right to ask that question.

Honestly, with all the paperwork that patients have to fill out, fax in, email over, or sign physically during their appointments, the informed consent form can feel like just another piece of paper. When you sign an informed consent form, for whatever procedure, appointment, test you are about to complete, you are acknowledging that you fully understand every risk involved, every benefit, all the possible outcomes of the intervention, and any alternatives, as well as giving your permission to move forward. You are explicitly stating that you have all the information available to you, you have reviewed it, have weighed your options, and have made the decision to move forward.

That changes the tone a little bit of the importance of informed consent, doesn't it?

If you are not well informed about the nuances of every aspect of your care, you can't make a good decision and actively participate in your healthcare because you don't have all the information you need at your disposal.

The foundations of informed consent

Optimally, open, detailed, and thorough conversations should happen between you and your care team about all the risks, benefits, alternatives, outcomes, and purposes of any intervention. Only after this conversation should you sign, or acknowledge, the informed consent.

A standard informed consent form has a fundamental framework that includes many of the following elements:

- **Complete explanation of the procedure:** Healthcare providers must provide to you the important and relevant information about the proposed intervention. In so many terms, this is an acknowledgement of key information (such as what the intervention will achieve, any risks, any complications involved in the administration of it, and possible outcomes of forgoing it).

  TIP

  Be sure to talk these details over with your care team. If you feel like you're only being presented with the positive benefits of an intervention and not the risks, or you don't have all the information about what not moving forward with a treatment would look like, for example, ask those questions before you sign anything. You don't want to find yourself in a position in which you signed off on something without having all the information.

- **Assurance that you understand the information presented:** Having the information is one thing, understanding it is something completely different. That's one reason why consent forms are written in what is referred to as simple language — they avoid medical jargon and the unfamiliar verbiage of the healthcare field to ensure that patients understand the information.
- **Freedom to make your own decision about proceeding essentially means that no one is pressuring you to do anything:** Sometimes patients feel like they have to make a certain decision or move forward with a certain course of action because they believe it will please their care team, their family, their friends, or someone other than themselves.

Your health is yours, and only yours. Conversations, decisions, interventions, and anything else pertaining to your health need to be acceptable in your eyes, even if other people around you are in opposition. You cannot be comfortable with a decision that you did not fully make, especially when you're the principal party affected by its outcomes.

WARNING

Some decisions take time to make. There is nothing wrong with taking the time that you need to gather more information about a decision, ask more questions, get other perspectives, or do whatever you need to do to be comfortable before making a decision.

If you are in an environment, such as during a clinical appointment, where you are feeling rushed to make a decision, it's your responsibility to respectfully and firmly state that you would like to take some time to fully consider the course of action.

More times than not, care teams are understanding and happy to respect your need to think decisions through thoroughly. If for some reason you are still being rushed or feeling coerced to make a specific decision, it's your responsibility and your right to remove yourself from the situation and revisit the conversation with people you trust, even if that means not working with the professional who pressured you.

» **Assurance that you can decide for yourself:** If the patient is unable to understand their options, ask questions about benefits and risks, or perform other functions to ensure that they can decide for themselves, individuals — such as a guardian or a power of attorney, who a patient may have appointed to make decisions on their behalf — can consider these factors for them and make a decision. People with significant disabilities, minors, elderly individuals, or individuals with conditions that affect their cognition may have their informed consent reviewed and signed by individuals who have the legal power to do so.

After reviewing all the key elements of an informed consent, having appropriate conversations with your care team to answer all your questions, and considering all the factors on the table, you can make an informed decision.

WARNING

By the time you sign the consent form, your decision should be clear. Be sure to identify any unclear points before you sign the form. Your signature, or verbal consent, is proof that you've done your homework and made your decision. The informed consent can also help manage expectations between you and your care providers so that there aren't misunderstandings down the road.

Legal implications of informed consent

Not only does the informed consent process satisfy ethical obligations of healthcare in empowering patients to make informed decisions, it also satisfies the legal requirements of the health system to ensure that there is proof that you made an informed decision about your treatments, medications, or procedures. While the informed consent process can safeguard your patient rights, it also protects the healthcare system from legal disputes and trouble.

Consider this scenario:

Adam is a concert pianist who has been working with his care team to identify ways to manage the debilitating symptoms of his chronic health condition.

After months of research, his provider suggests that he undergo a series of newly developed treatments that can reduce the severity of his symptoms and get him back to his idea of normal. Adam is excited to finally find an option that could present some promise, so he signs the consent form without asking questions about the side-effects of the treatment.

After completing a couple treatments, he notices that the dexterity in his fingers had been affected and he begins having trouble playing the piano the way he used to. Devastated by this observation, he does some research about the side-effects of the treatments he's been taking and notices that the symptoms he's been experiencing are a risk common to the treatment.

Furious about this observation, Adam decides to take up legal action against the hospital. He is then presented with the consent form that he signed, agreeing to the procedure and risk, which outlined the potential side-effects he could experience, including the one that he had.

Adam's experience went sideways and led to a very distressing situation for him. Can you spot the opportunities Adam had to learn about the impact of the treatment he was about to endure?

If Adam claimed that he was not properly informed about the risk of the treatment and experienced harm and did not sign an informed consent, the conversation from a legal aspect may be different. If Adam would have had conversations about the risks and benefits of the treatment with his care team, he could have become aware of the potential side-effect he experienced. Determining whether the benefits of the intervention outweigh the risks is a personal decision. Since Adam is a pianist, this may have been a deal breaker for him — we can't know this since he was not aware of these side-effects.

If you have questions about your patient rights from a legal perspective or about more nuanced issues regarding informed consent, consult with a licensed attorney to identify necessary steps and precautions you may need to take.

REMEMBER

Don't stay up all night wondering what could or could not go wrong after you have signed a consent form. If you approach the informed consent process conversation with your care team with the goal of fully understanding the considerations and risks, you will be able to make a decision that you can stand behind. And, if for some reason you make a decision and then change your mind, you can work with your clinical care team to make the appropriate adjustments regarding that intervention.

Informed consent and patient autonomy

You may have heard of a field of study called *ethics*. Broadly, the ethics of a discipline, like medicine, is concerned with the ideology of good and bad. In medical and bioethics, the principle of autonomy, or a person's ability to make their own decision about matters that affect them, is a good thing.

To be an autonomous patient not only means that you have the freedom to be as present in your care as you want to be, it also affords you the opportunity to, within the realm of competence, call the shots about your own healthcare. Informed consent is a catalyst for patient autonomy.

When you make a decision about your care, you are affirming your autonomy to make a decision about what you want to happen to you and your body.

Healthcare providers want patients to participate in treatments, activities, and conversations that are in their best interest and that will reduce the possibility of causing harm.

To identify if something is in your best interest, you have to have all the information about what could happen, which ties back into the presentation of information.

Understanding Your Role in Informed Consent

Now that you know that the informed consent process can protect your power as a patient and can serve as a tool to make sure that you properly understand all aspects of any medical intervention, it's important to understand that you also have responsibilities.

Controlling the narrative

The following lists outlines some important things you should be doing to ensure that you are well positioned to make an informed decision, *prior* to signing an informed consent form.

1. **Talk to your healthcare providers about the intervention or treatment.**

   Members of your care team should make an intentional effort to have a conversation with you about all relevant factors pertaining to the intervention. That includes explaining the function of the intervention, what it aims to do, its benefits and risks, how it will affect your condition (and what the diagnosis or condition is), alternatives, what you can expect to gain from the treatment, and what might happen if you don't do anything.

   Take notes or create a checklist to address your questions. Your providers may use a variety of educational tools, like handouts or videos, to relay this information to you in a way that is easy for you to digest. Some providers show you diagrams or other visual tools to help you understand.

   REMEMBER

   This conversation should take as long as you need it to. If you are uncomfortable or unsure about a specific part of the information, you have the right to work with your clinical care team and gain a better understanding. If that means you need to go back and revisit information from earlier, do it.

2. **Take your time digesting the information and ask questions that you feel are necessary to clarify your understanding.**

   A good care team will expect and anticipate questions. Chances are, you're on this journey for the first time, even if you are revisiting certain parts of your journey again. There is often a lot to consider when making a decision about your health.

   If, while listening to your clinical team's presentation, you don't have an answer to one or more of your questions, feel free to politely ask your provider directly to answer it. Say something like "Thanks for letting me know the benefits of this medication, but could you tell me about the side effects I could experience in taking it?" or "What can I expect this treatment to do for my condition?" By asking specific, direct questions like these, you give your clinical team the opportunity to provide a streamlined, direct answer.

   Don't allow yourself to feel rushed or become self-conscious about taking too much time to think through the questions you have. Whatever time it takes for you to be comfortable making a decision is the time it takes, period. In cases outside of emergency medical treatment, you have time to weigh all your pros and cons before a treatment or intervention begins.

TIP

Sometimes, clinical providers may need to administer emergency interventions to save your life. If you have strong feelings about the use of blood products, transfusions, resuscitation attempts, and more, make sure your wishes are reflected in an *advance directive,* which is explored in Chapter 18. Advance directives and living wills communicate your wishes in the event you're unable to make an informed decision yourself. Be sure to complete one and make sure it's accessible in the event of emergency. Without them, lifesaving treatments will be administered without your permission.

3. **Be honest with your care team about any concerns you have.**

   As you are presented with information, you may hear about risks, adverse reactions, or outcomes that concern you. It's important to be honest with your team if you are uncomfortable with any component of the treatment.

   Ask yourself if you are uncomfortable with certain aspects of the plan because you don't know enough about them or just don't like or find comfort in the plan. As awesome as healthcare providers are, they are not mind readers.

   It's your responsibility to make these things known to them. When you share your concerns, you open a door with your team to further reassess if the proposed treatment or intervention is the best one for you.

   You can have a brainstorming session to find or refine the plan that makes the most sense for you — but it all starts with you being honest and voicing your concerns.

4. **Let your team know if you need accommodations or additional resources to help you with the informed consent process.**

   You should have the tools you need to comfortably gather the appropriate information, ask questions, and make an informed decision about your care, regardless of the challenges you navigate. If you need an informed consent form in a different language, or a form with a larger print or another accessibility function, ask for it. If your care team does not have appropriate resources, ask them to find them.

If you feel like you are being bothersome by asking for accommodations, it may be a good idea to contact the hospital ombudsman or the department for disability accommodations.

5. **Don't rely on dialogue; physically review your consent form.**

   Yes, that means actually reading it. Since you will be signing or acknowledging and consenting to the terms of the informed consent agreement, it's in your best interest to read it — just like you would any other document you sign. Having a conversation with your care team about the particulars of an intervention is important; however, this shouldn't be the only information review you have.

   Review the document to make sure that you understand everything that's in it. In conversation, the care team member could have forgotten to mention something written in the consent or may have misspoke.

Communicating effectively

As in any part of your healthcare journey, grasping what you want to communicate, how you need to communicate it, and how to ensure you're understood are all crucial to the success of your patient self-advocacy efforts.

In addition to asking questions and advocating for resources to allow you to make an informed decision, make sure that your communication throughout the entire process is streamlined and simple. Consider these tips to communicate effectively during the informed consent process:

» **Repeat back, or teach back, what you understand to your care team.** By repeating what you hear and understand, you allow your clinical care team to clarify, provide additional information if needed, and possibly correct any misunderstandings.

  As a call to action for your efforts, you can end the summary of what you've heard and understood with a statement such as, "Did I understand this the way I was intended to?" or "Is there anything I am misunderstanding?"

  You should also communicate what you understand is required of you in the next steps. If you are comfortable with the information, the next steps could be for you to sign the consent form and schedule your treatment. If you are not comfortable, your next steps could be seeing additional providers that can give you more information about the intervention.

» **Intentionally communicate how parts of the process make you feel.** If you are feeling overwhelmed or uncomfortable with the information, plainly state that. This is not the time to be nuanced and mysterious. Your clinical care team wants to understand how you're feeling, what about the process is making you feel that way, and what they can do about it. You can say things like, "I'm not very clear on the risks of this treatment and am feeling overwhelmed because of that; can we go back to that section and review again?" or "I'm not sure if this treatment plan is the best option for me, but I would like to revisit the part of the conversation about alternative treatments. Can you give me additional information about that?"

  By communicating your feelings clearly, the component that's making you feel a certain way, and what you need to move forward, you take the guesswork out for your care team out and position them to further the conversation in a direction that is most meaningful to you.

» **Listen actively to the information that's being presented.** When you're going through the informed consent process, your full attention needs to be on the conversation with your provider and the consent in front of you. Minimize multitasking.

  Just because you have questions doesn't mean that you weren't listening. Sometimes information from your care team is not presented as plainly as you may need. However, approach these conversations with your full attention, not scrolling through social media, completing tasks that can be done afterwards, or having conversations with other people who are not related to the consent process.

  If you're having trouble hearing the person who is performing the informed consent or concentrating on what they're saying, it's okay to ask other people in the room to lower their voices, allow you the opportunity to think, or even leave the room. People who are truly supportive of your empowerment as a patient won't mind.

Recognizing Common Challenges with Consent

The goal of the informed consent process is to ensure that a patient has access to and understands all the information regarding a treatment. It presents patients with the opportunity to make a decision in the best interest of their care. The tricky thing is, additional considerations during the consent process can make it challenging.

For patients whose primary or native language is not the language that their healthcare providers speaks, patients with different cultural or religious backgrounds, those with cognitive impairments, such as intellectual disabilities, or those with health literacy challenges, the informed consent process may not be so straightforward. In this section, you learn about some of the common challenges with consent, review a few real-world examples, and are presented with a few recommendations to address those challenges.

Written versus verbal consent

A patient can provide informed consent through their written signature, or verbally, using their words. The printed informed consent form asks for a written expression of your informed consent.

Usually, more complex or invasive procedures require written acknowledgement of informed consent, unless there is a physical reason that the patient can't sign (like having a broken hand or being doubled over in pain). In many cases, written consent is the "cleanest," because the consent form is very easy to document and produce. It provides a thorough outline of all components of the treatment, and it can provide a paper trail for legal and ethical protection.

Verbal consent is also an acceptable form of informed consent. This is when you verbally agree to understanding all aspects of the treatment or intervention you are being presented with and have made an informed decision to move forward. Verbal consent is often used with routine procedures, such as when your clinician explains the process of checking your blood glucose levels in the office and asks if you are okay with proceeding.

In both types of consent, you express your agreement to take the proposed action; however, each form has its strengths and weaknesses. Written consents may be the easiest to document, but they are often full of medical terminology that patients are not familiar with and may struggle to navigate. Some patients feel pressured to sign on the dotted line as a formality and are not afforded the opportunity to start a conversation.

Although verbal consent is relatively quick and catalyzed by dialogue with a healthcare provider, it can be difficult to document. Patients have to rely on the information shared with them verbally to make a decision, and there may be pressure to say yes, especially when it's a relatively low-risk procedure.

To improve the written and verbal consent process from a patient perspective, make sure that your provider walks you through each point on the written consent. For verbal consent, it's important to give yourself time to make an appropriate decision. You can slow down the pace of the consent process in both cases, to ensure you fully understand the information that's being presented.

Digital communication consent

Technology has become a central modality and partner in the provision of healthcare, specifically when it comes to telehealth. With virtual visits (an more often now, in-person visits), it's becoming more common for patients to review consent forms electronically, either through their online health management app or by using a secure patient portal. This potentially easier consent offering doesn't come without some unique challenges.

For some patients, being sent an electronic consent form can feel cold because there isn't a person in front of them to answer any questions they have (see Figure 4-1).

For individuals who are not tech-savvy, understanding how to navigate platforms, such as video chats and portals, can be challenging. Patients may also have questions and concerns about their private information being on electronic platforms, even when they are secure and encrypted.

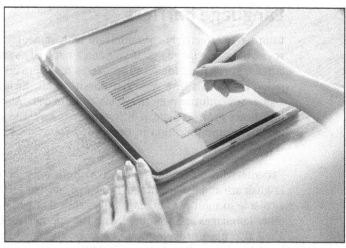

maruco/Getty Images

FIGURE 4-1: The electronic consent form can feel cold and uncaring to some.

While technology can make some patients' journeys easier, it can also pose barriers to the following:

- Some elderly patients
- Patients who don't feel comfortable utilizing technology
- Patients who have limited access to the Internet

Even though the healthcare industry is evolving at the speed of technology, there are real implications and necessary safeguards that need to be put in place to ensure that patients feel just as comfortable, supported, and informed when submitting a consent form digitally as they are in person.

TIP

If you are uncomfortable utilizing a digital consent form, reach out to your provider's office and ask if there is a way for you to do your informed consent in person or on a physical document that can be mailed to you.

REMEMBER

Review all the information on a digital consent form just as carefully as you would a paper copy. It may be tempting to click through the pages and hit the acknowledgement button at the end of the form because it's on a screen, and not on a piece of paper in front of you with a provider.

Language barriers

In order to effectively communicate with someone, you need to speak the same language. If you don't naturally speak the same language, you need tools and resources to ensure accurate translation of content in a way that doesn't omit, include, or make vague any information that was unintended. Although many healthcare providers speak different languages, the primary language of communication in the United States healthcare system is English.

Patients who have limited English proficiency or don't speak English are at a disadvantage. Informed consent forms should be available in multiple languages to ensure that patients speaking other languages are presented with the appropriate information. They also need to have their questions answered in a language in which they're fluent. If you feel like you are navigating a language barrier in your healthcare journey because you do not fluently speak English, look for professional translation services available from your health system. If they are not offered, ask for an interpreter.

REMEMBER

Many patients who do not speak English feel the need to bring a friend or a family member with them to translate. Although this support can be helpful, the health system has a responsibility to provide professional translation services by trained translators who understand medical terminology. Patients should not have to solve these communication barriers on their own.

TIP

Ask your care team to add a note to your medical record about your preferred language. This may reduce the downtime you might experience waiting for language support and can also be helpful in emergencies, when communication must happen as soon as possible.

Cultural and religious considerations

Cultural and religious beliefs sometimes impact the way that a patient understands and approaches the informed consent process. Western healthcare culture often advocates for individual autonomy, where patients are empowered to make their own informed decisions about their own healthcare. However in other cultures, it may be common for patients to collectively make decisions with members of their support system, such as elders in their community.

If there are cultural or religious considerations that are important to you and are relevant to the informed consent process, be sure to let your care team know what they are and explain how they can respect your wishes.

Of course, you don't owe anyone an explanation about what you believe, where you come from, and what's important to you. However, it is your responsibility to make your care team aware so that you reduce the probability of them being disrespectful or dismissive. Although cultural sensitivity and continuing education about cultural and religious differences is often a core part of the hospital employee professional development curriculum, don't assume that people know.

TIP

If you feel uncomfortable having to explain certain religious or cultural differences to your care team, consider bringing an advocate who can help.

It may feel like you are relinquishing some of your power to explain to someone else why you do things differently because you have different beliefs or come from different places. However, educating your care team will make you more empowered as a patient.

REMEMBER

If you feel weird or uncomfortable about educating people who do not share your same cultural or religious beliefs about yours, remember why you are doing it. You are sharing information about your human experience that could ultimately affect the quality of care you receive.

2

Mastering Communication with Healthcare Professionals

IN THIS PART . . .

Developing effective and respectful communication with your clinical care team

Coming prepared to your appointments with the right questions and the best approach to maximize your time with your clinician

IN THIS CHAPTER

» Clearly defining team roles and care objectives

» Encouraging transparent interactions

» Leveraging technology for better communication

» Using your emotional intelligence to build bridges

» Cultivating collaborative decision-making

Chapter 5
Cultivating Mutually Respectful Relationships with Your Care Team

Any relationship worth having takes work. Whether it's a romantic relationship, a great friendship, or even a care-giving relationship with your favorite pet (or pets — the more the merrier!), it takes time, patience, understanding, trust, empathy, and accountability. Your relationship with your clinician and clinical team is no different. Your clinical care team should be your go-to group of people to help you problem-solve and navigate the complexities of your healthcare. Your relationship should foster a sense of openness, urgency, and initiative that continuously pulls all relevant team members together to game plan the next moves of your healthcare journey.

By cultivating a collaborative, trusting relationship with your clinician and care team, you set yourself up to handle whatever comes your way as a unit on a shared mission. Each perspective is recognized and valued as you appraise symptoms, review diagnoses, navigate treatment options, and maintain and improve your health and well-being. The bottom line is that you get out of the relationship what you put into it.

In this chapter, you learn how to implement open communication channels, establish clear expectations of your care team, learn techniques for nurturing solid and trusting relationships, and consider ways to foster collaborative decision-making. I teach you how to get the most out of your relationship with your clinician by respecting them, and I educate you on how they need to respect you.

TIP

An important part of being respectful of your healthcare team is being respectful of their time. Try your best to make it to your appointments on time and if you're unable to do so, give the office a call in advance or reschedule your appointment. Practices like this ensure that everyone using the healthcare system has the opportunity to use it efficiently.

Building Open Communication Channels

People who communicate well are more likely to be successful in everything they do because they know how to articulate their thoughts and feelings about a subject clearly, prompt others to confess their thoughts, and clarify even the most confusing topics. Communication is a critical component in having a good relationship with your clinician. Only some clinician are good communicators; the same could be said for patients navigating the healthcare system.

When communication is solid, little to no information is left up to interpretation. The listener doesn't have to make assumptions about what the speaker means, and the objectives are clear. If you are serious about taking charge of your health and navigating the healthcare system triumphantly, you can't afford to take a chance on spotty communication. Lack of communication can contribute to misunderstandings, medical errors, patient safety concerns, subpar medical care, and the deterioration of a positive relationship with your clinician.

So, you get it — communication is essential. But how do you ensure that you communicate correctly and efficiently with your clinician and other clinical care team members? The hospital has hundreds of telephone extensions, it takes forever to get a response from your provider's office by email, and it can feel like sending a fax to the office is like throwing a dart at a board in the middle of the night and hoping for a bull's eye. This section explains how to set clear communication expectations with your care team, use technological resources to get the job done, and make your voice heard.

Establishing an effective communication feedback system

Effective communication between you and your care team is a dynamic interplay of proactive and reactive approaches. Here's the breakdown. Initiating a strategy to communicate with your care team — by outlining your goals for communicating relevant information, setting your expectations, and detailing your preferred methods of support — is a proactive step. This helps ensure that everyone knows what communication should look like from the start. Your communication strategy should also be reactive — a flexible process that evolves and improves with feedback from you and your clinical team. Consider this example:

At an appointment with her new primary care physician, Kendra shared with her clinician that she would like to receive communication about her test results through the hospital's online health management tool (like MyChart) as soon as they became available. Her clinician takes note of her communication expectations, and she starts receiving her test results through that platform. Over the next month, she realizes that she is having issues staying logged into the online health management tool and has missed some communication from her clinician. Before her next office visit, she calls the office and explains that she would like to receive a phone call from the doctor's office when her test results are available through the online health management tool while she figures out what's going on with her login access.

Kendra's initial communication to her clinician that she wanted communication about her test results to come through the health management tool was proactive. She was upfront about her preferences and gained her provider's support and agreement to follow that communication plan. Her communication was also reactive, in that she provided feedback when she experienced technical difficulties accessing the health management tool and asked her clinician to call her when an update was available. She recognized the issue, made her care team aware, proposed an alternative communication solution that allowed her to access the needed information, and gained her clinician's buy-in (and action) to support it.

Large organizations utilize communication feedback systems to gather consumer feedback and response data so they can improve their products or services (hospitals even use them to collect patient experience data — you may know them as surveys). Since you are a consumer of the service your healthcare team provides, you must set up your own communication feedback system with your providers.

By setting up feedback systems for different components of your clinical care, you will have a crystal-clear plan for the following:

- What you're communicating to which parties
- Why you're communicating it
- How that communication will occur
- The questions that communication needs to address
- The methods utilized to gather this information
- How you will adjust the system as you receive feedback
- How you will act on the feedback you receive

Building a patient self-advocacy feedback system

You can navigate your healthcare like a pro by implementing a patient self-advocacy feedback system. In a notebook, online document, or note on your phone, build a feedback system for different aspects of your care journey to share with your clinical care team as you manage expectations as a group.

Consider this scenario:

Tom and his doctor decide to start a new medication to manage symptoms of his chronic health condition that had stopped responding to the medication he had been taking for a couple of years. He is open to trying a new medication but is nervous about the possibility of experiencing side-effects that his doctor outlined. Before he leaves the doctor's office, he asks for a foolproof plan for handling the presentation of side-effects, if he experiences any, and how they will work with him to identify the next course of treatment.

WARNING

Listen very closely and ensure you understand the potential side-effects of any new or existing treatment plan. Ask your clinician how you should respond. Always follow your clinician's advice when reporting or seeking emergency medical treatment if you experience potentially life-threatening or harmful side-effects — before you use any other communication tools or techniques.

Here's how you build a feedback system to communicate with your clinician and clinical care team:

1. **Identify your objectives for the communication.**

   Ask yourself, "What am I trying to communicate?" "Who needs to know this information?" Why do they need to know it?" You are communicating your reaction or experience to your clinician. You should also ask yourself what you expect to gain from submitting feedback to your clinician. You can gain further insights about your response to the medication that will help drive your decision-making.

2. **Choose your methods for providing feedback.**

   Establish which modalities, platforms, and tools you will use to communicate this information to your clinician. Some examples could be using an online health management tool, like MyChart, calling the office, sending an email, or scheduling a follow-up appointment.

   TIP

   Use a communication method that is easy and intuitive for you and your care team.

3. **Pinpoint the questions your feedback answers for your provider.**

   Impactful feedback should clearly and concisely answer a predefined set of questions the recipient wants to answer. Your feedback on a new treatment option should answer questions for your provider like "Is the patient tolerating this treatment well?" or "Are they experiencing any side effects?" to name a few. This will help you streamline your communication to what's relevant and reduce the probability of rambling (after all, you and your clinician want to get to the facts).

4. **Put your system in motion.**

   Your communication feedback system is only helpful if you use it! After hammering out the details, use the system to engage your care team. Putting the system into motion shows your clinician and your clinical team that you are actively involved in your healthcare and you recognize the importance of communicating with them.

   TIP

   It's helpful to summarize the critical points of your feedback system to your clinical team. For example, if you plan to submit feedback about a new medication, tell your clinician, "Thanks for the information. I will let you know how the new medication works via MyChart message to support our collaborative decision-making about the best course of treatment for my condition. The goal of my feedback is to let you know how I'm tolerating the medication, how it impacts my daily routine, and my ability to afford it".

5. **Note your system's effectiveness and make changes when necessary.**

   It's important to remember that communication systems are dynamic — they need to react to the current environment and evolve. Keep an eye out for parts of your system that continue to work and those that don't. Encourage conversations with your provider and ask their opinion. Hopefully, it will be impactful for you too.

   REMEMBER

   Constructive criticism is helpful on both sides of the proverbial bedrail. Be kind to yourself. Build and make changes to your feedback system. When you receive honest feedback from your care team that there is room for improvement, take it as a win. You started the conversation and are in the driver's seat of your care. No one is expecting you to be perfect!

6. **Make your feedback actionable.**

   Now that you have all this great feedback, it's your responsibility to make sure your clinical team uses it to improve your care, make evidence-based decisions alongside you about your care, facilitate relevant conversations about your feedback, and make sure your insights are noted in your medical records, especially if they are regarding your experience with a treatment option or plan.

Think of your communication feedback system as a loop, because it has no end. As you move through different phases of your care, welcome more members of your care team, and evolve as a patient, you will need new strategies to communicate about each aspect of your care. Over time, you will find a sweet spot in a communication system and will be able to "plug and chug" any new information into it and experience repeated success.

You can also take advantage of the patient feedback offerings at your hospital, such as filling out the patient experience and engagement surveys emailed to you after a clinician's visit. Providing insight into your experience in the health system lets hospital leadership know what's working from your perspective and what needs improvement. Usually, you're not asked to provide personal information. You simply fill out a few multiple-choice questions and an optional extended response about your experience. Good clinical providers and healthcare workers want to know what part of their healthcare offering is helpful to the patient and what needs work.

TIP

Prioritize sending an email now and then or requesting a brief meeting with some of your regular clinical team members to discuss their performance and support of your care and identify areas for improvement. In the spirit of collaborative improvement, ask them what you can do to make their job easier as well.

REMEMBER

All your communication systems don't have to look the same. It may make sense to communicate feedback by telephone for certain parts of your care, while in other cases, it makes sense to take pictures and attach them to a MyChart message. Don't be afraid to mix and match options to find the best strategies.

Encouraging clinical team dialogue and participation

I'm sure you've heard the saying, "It takes a village to raise a child." It also takes a village to support a patient and ensure they get the health outcomes they seek. If you haven't experienced it already, you will have to work with many healthcare professionals along your journey through the healthcare system to get you where you need to go. It's helpful to think of this never-ending roster of people as members of your team.

Each member has a different role and responsibility to ensure you're supported. Each member's perspective is valuable and insightful. But what happens when some team members are overly active and maybe even dominate the conversation, while others seem to be passengers?

Spoiler alert — when the communication isn't balanced and collaborative, you as the patient probably won't get:

- The support you deserve
- The outcomes you seek
- All the relevant information to make an informed decision
- The guarantee that you won't rip your hair out in frustration

REMEMBER

A key component to feeling respected is feeling safe and encouraged to provide your input and perspective without fear of dismissal or judgment. You want that as a patient, and your care team wants that as a support partner.

The following tips can help encourage dialogue and participation from your clinical care team:

- **Create an inclusive environment where everyone feels heard and valued:** Two (or more!) heads are better than one when collecting information, weighing the pros and cons, and putting a plan together. As the patient and the consumer of the system, the final word is yours; however, you can create an environment where the perspective of your nurse is just as important as the perspective of your clinician or social worker, or any other member of your team. They may have different specializations, but they work together to support you. You can say things like, "I'd love to hear your perspective" or "Is there anything I should consider from a [*insert discipline here*] standpoint?"
- **Encourage open-ended questions during the discussion:** Don't settle for "yes" or "no" responses from your team. Ask questions that prompt them to answer questions without limitations. Instead of asking, "Have you heard back from orthopedics yet?" ask, "What information are we waiting on from orthopedics?" Your team then has an opportunity to provide a more robust response.

» **Be present and attentive when they are speaking:** Honestly, this is just good manners. If you were speaking to someone, and they weren't actively engaged in what you had to say, scrolling through their phone while trying to make a point, odds are you wouldn't feel very valued. Extend the same courtesy to every member of your care team.

TIP

You can still be attentive and present in conversations with your providers while taking notes about what they are saying. This is entirely different from watching Facebook videos of a cat eating peanut butter while your discharge nurse is trying to review your medication list. By all means, watch the video (it's probably hilarious), but do it after your nurse leaves the room.

» **Remember to say "thank you" when someone goes above and beyond for you:** Clinical care teams have responsibilities to their patients to keep them safe, administer proper treatment, and improve their well-being. But it's not just about their duties; it's about the people behind those duties. So, take a moment to recognize the humanity in the care you receive and thank your team for their support. Make sure you extend this gratitude to anyone who makes your experience better — like the front desk scheduler who was able to get you a same-day appointment on a day you were feeling really sick — and don't just reserve this courtesy for your clinician. This is a team effort.

REMEMBER

It pays dividends to make sure that everyone who is supporting your care feels appreciated and able to provide their insights so you can make an informed decision about your care. However, it is imperative that they extend the same courtesy to you. You have the right to be treated fairly, listened to, and encouraged to provide your input in decision making.

Using technology to improve communication

Technology presents endless applications in the healthcare system. Every other day, there is a new fitness app to download, a health-tracking watch to buy, and a dashboard to review so you can organize your current medications. Technological tools are there to make it easier to communicate with clinician. Fifty years ago, I'm sure no one would have thought that you could sit in front of a camera and have a face-to-face conversation with your doctor whose office is 60 minutes from your house!

You can use technology like videoconferencing (such as Microsoft Teams, FaceTime, and Zoom), secure messaging apps, and more to enhance communication with your care team. Technology can make it easier to communicate with your care team, especially when you:

» Need a virtual visit
» Need to share pictures or medical records
» Are on the go and need to send a quick message to your team without calling the office

TIP

Ask your doctor's office which tech tools they use to help improve communication. Not all hospitals use the same systems, so you can streamline your options by asking what's available. You can also ask for training or help guides using the online health management portal, video conferencing platform, or data-sharing technologies. If you're unfamiliar with your hospital's tech communication tools, you won't be able to use them effectively. See Appendix A for much more about using technology effectively.

Establishing Clear Expectations

Laying the ground rules and managing expectations of your relationship with your care team, in the beginning, sets you up for success down the road.

Imagine playing a new board game. As excited as you are to jump in with your friends and start playing the game, you know that it would be helpful to read the instructions because they outline the game's roles, responsibilities, and rules. When you understand these components, you know how each player should interact with the game and with each other. Without this information, it's the Wild, Wild West.

Someone could be accused of cheating in the middle of the game, but no one can substantiate that claim because no one knows the rules — the same goes for relationships. When you understand your place in the relationship, what to expect, and what is expected of you, everyone in the relationship can maintain accountability and can understand what your support and involvement looks like.

Identifying team roles and responsibilities

The roles and responsibilities of a patient and a provider can be lengthy; however, this section covers some universal expectations.

As a patient, you must be:

- Respectful to your provider and all those around you
- An active participant in your own healthcare
- Honest with your provider
- Knowledgeable of your financial responsibility to your medical care and the health system
- Willing to work collaboratively with key stakeholders in your clinical and medical care
- Aware of your rights as a patient
- Knowledgeable of and observant of hospital rules and regulations
- Empowered to make decisions about your healthcare

This is in no way an exhaustive list; however, these responsibilities certainly make the highlight reel.

TIP

You can ask your providers their opinion on what makes for a good working relationship with the patient. From their feedback, you can review your list of rules and responsibilities and add components accordingly.

Your clinical team providers have the responsibility to:

- Place the patient at the center of their healthcare and provide as personalized a form of medicine as possible to treat conditions
- Diagnose and treat medical conditions
- Prioritize prevention as well as treat illness and injury
- Educate patients

» Provide scientific, evidence-based solutions for disease treatment
» Keep patient information confidential and abide by privacy laws
» Keep accurate medical records

Again, not an exhaustive list, but you should get the picture.

TIP

If you have questions about what services or support your providers should offer you, ask them directly. If you don't feel comfortable asking your personal care team, you can request general patient information from other departments in the hospital. They can give you a basic overview of the roles and responsibilities of some of the members of your team.

There will, no doubt, be other members of your care team that you will work with on a daily basis, including nurses, social workers, front desk staff, care coordinators, patient advocates, and more. It's important that, as you get to know these individuals, you get in the habit of asking them what they do and how their role supports patient care. By having this conversation, you increase your repertoire of knowledge of the support and can manage your expectations.

WARNING

If you suspect that a member of your care team is not functioning within the parameters of their roles and responsibilities, and you feel that your care is being compromised, you may want to have a clarifying conversation with that member. If you feel that the care you are receiving is unethical, the treatment is inappropriate, or you are being placed at risk, work with your hospital ombudsman office or a private patient advocate to resolve the situation.

Setting achievable goals

Setting achievable goals is critical to your care. It helps slowly build momentum toward the outcome you want to see. Identifying "bite-sized" wins is a great way to ensure your treatment plans are actionable and within reach.

Goals that are *SMART* (specific, measurable, achievable, relevant, and time-bound — see Chapter 7) are more achievable. For example:

UNDERSTANDING YOUR RIGHTS AND RESPONSIBILITIES AS A PATIENT

Knowing your rights as a patient and your responsibilities to yourself and to the collaborative efforts of your care team is the cornerstone of patient empowerment. As cheesy as it sounds, knowledge is power, and not knowing your rights can be detrimental to the success of your healthcare navigation.

Hospitals have a responsibility to inform patients of their rights, or the protections that are allotted to them as they received care. If you haven't been presented with a list of patient rights, ask for them. Some of your key patient rights include these:

- You have the right to receive the highest standard of care.
- You have the right to be treated with respect.
- You have the right to be presented with comprehensive information about any treatment or intervention so that you can make an informed decision.
- You have the right to access your medical records.
- You have the right to privacy of your sensitive and important information, like your Social Security Number, health information, and so on. If you want to share this information with anyone, you have the right to sign a release form.
- You have the right to seek emergency medical treatment, even if you can't afford it.
- You have the right to make decisions about your healthcare, including the refusal of treatment.

Although this is not an exhaustive list of patient rights, these are some of the highlights. Familiarize yourself with patient rights at your hospital.

Angie wants to cut her A1C (a measure of blood sugar related to diabetes) to less than 7 percent in the next nine months by modifying her diet, losing 25 pounds, and taking the insulin her doctor has prescribed to her.

This is a SMART goal because it's specific, can be measured, is achievable, and has a time commitment attached to it.

TIP

BEST PRACTICES FOR COMMUNICATING WITH YOUR CARE TEAM

Here are some tips for communicating like a pro with your care team:

- **Be kind when you communicate:** I don't know about you, but I don't make it a habit of going the extra mile for people who go out of their way to speak to me nastily (maybe one day I will, but I'm not there yet). Your care team can help make your healthcare experience overly positive. Treat people the way you would like to be treated.
- **Ask for confirmation when you can:** If you talk to someone over the phone and they give you instructions, set an appointment, or fill a prescription, ask for confirmation to be sent to your email, mailed home, or posted on your electronic health management portal so you can remember what they said or did and have record of the communication.
- **Know your medical record number (MRN):** If you have a common name (like me), it can be easy for your care team to pull up the wrong patient account. Learn your MRN number and securely confirm it when scheduling appointments, filling medications, and performing other healthcare duties.

  Your MRN is sensitive information and protected under HIPAA, so protect it and don't throw it around willy-nilly.
- **Prepare your questions before office visits:** Spend time thinking about what you want to ask your clinician, what information is important to relay, and what questions you have before the appointment. This way you can hit the ground running and don't have to spend time (and frustration) trying to remember what you wanted to ask.
- **Be observant of office business hours relative to emergency situations:** You're not going to have much luck getting in contact with anyone at your doctor's office calling ten minutes before they close for the day. Plan to make routine, non-urgent communication to your providers during office hours and familiarize yourself with emergency services contact information, in the event you need immediate medical care.

You can ask your clinician who to call when you experience certain situations. They will tell you when you need to call 911, go to urgent care, or schedule an office visit. Your safety is their number one priority.

- **Create a "elevator pitch" of your healthcare journey to share at new and established health visits:** As much as providers would like to spend hours with you reviewing your symptoms and recent health events, appointment are only so long. Highlight the key points you want to touch on and practice communicating them in a matter of minutes. If your provider has questions, they will ask and you can utilize the limited appointment time more efficiently.

Once you've defined what you want to achieve, a partnership with your clinical care team is imperative. Talk with your clinician about where to start. Engage them in conversations and brainstorm to discuss how to achieve your SMART goals.

You will find in this conversation an alignment between what you want to see and what your provider feels is clinically achievable.

Accessing Your Emotional Intelligence

Emotional intelligence is the ability to sense other people's feelings (along with your own) and recognize and manage emotions.

Being an emotionally intelligent member of society has its benefits, but being an emotionally intelligent consumer of the healthcare system gives you superpowers (you probably won't get x-ray vision, but you get my point). Becoming emotionally intelligent can lead to better clinical outcomes and less stress. Working with your clinical care team members empathetically and constructively can improve relationships with everyone involved.

How to be an emotionally intelligent patient

Taking charge of your health and being an active participant in your healthcare is undoubtedly a big responsibility, but a responsibility worth shouldering. Navigating the healthcare system can be challenging because there are things you don't know, pain and discomfort you might have to feel while trying to figure it out, as well as questions you might not have the answers to. The benefit of navigating the healthcare system with your clinical team is that you can foster a positive, collaborative relationship and they can help you get through the worst of it.

Here are some tips for being an emotionally intelligent patient:

- **Communicate your concerns and emotions in a calm, clear, respectful manner:** Every emotion that you feel on your healthcare journey is valid and your providers may benefit from knowing what they are. Take the initiative to communicate your emotions, your symptoms, and any other relevant information genuinely, clearly, and calmly. Even If you are experiencing negative emotions, you can convey them in a dignified manner. Practice saying things like "I'm feeling very overwhelmed with the information you're presenting me right now and it's giving me anxiety" or "The last time we spoke, I became angry because. . ."
- **Adopt a strategy to manage your emotions:** Everyone has emotions and it's normal to feel them, especially in conversations about health and quality of life. Work with a trusted healthcare provider, friend, or family member, or do your own research about how to regulate your emotions in a healthy way. Deep breathing exercises, yoga, time in nature, and journaling are some options to try.
- **Learn to practice patience:** Practicing patience doesn't mean waiting idly and not ensuring that progress is being made. It means that you understand that healthcare improvements, discoveries, diagnoses, and even getting on your clinician's schedule takes time. Your provider is likely working as quickly as they can to process imaging, get labs back, and follow up on your course of treatment.

  REMEMBER

  You can be patient but still hold your providers and clinical care team accountable for responding to your questions, following up on test results, and putting a plan of action together. Being patient doesn't mean being idle.
- **Show empathy to your clinician and your care team:** The flawed healthcare system presents multiple opportunities to improve the patient — and provider — experience. Your

clinician is human, which means they can experience stress, frustration, and fatigue, just like you. Show an understanding of their position, recognize their humanity, and make them feel valued as they help you navigate the healthcare maze.

TIP

Your support of their humanity doesn't remove your power as a patient to ensure you receive the support you need. Be understanding yet clear and purposeful about getting the care you need.

How to spot an emotionally intelligent provider

Ask yourself these questions to determine if your clinician or provider is emotionally intelligent:

- **Do they listen to you?** When you are conversing with your clinician about new symptoms, asking questions about a medication, or giving them an update on the events that have happened regarding your health, does your provider make eye contact with you? Do they listen to you without interrupting? Do they ask questions about what you've said? Do you feel like you don't have to repeat yourself multiple times? If not, they're probably not giving you their full attention.

  TIP

  Providers often have to type on their computers to document the conversation when they are talking to you. If you see them doing this, don't assume that they're not listening. Look for other signs of active listening, like eye contact, asking relevant questions in response to your story, and nodding as you speak.
- **Do they talk *to* you and not *at* you?** People who are not genuinely interested in the perspective of the other person they are "talking to" drone on and on about what they have to say and leave very little room for a response. An emotionally intelligent provider values communication and healthy dialogue. If you feel like you can't get a word in when talking to your clinician, you might have uncovered an emotional intelligence red flag.
- **Do they avoid "speaking doctor" to you?** Using plain or nonmedical language when communicating with a patient helps comprehension and retention of information. Your provider should realize that showing off their impressive

clinical vocabulary doesn't do you any favors; it just shows how out of touch they are.

- **Do they pay attention to your body language and other subtle cues when you're speaking with them?** Imagine you receive difficult news from your clinician, and they explain to you what to expect next. As they talk, you become extremely quiet and hyper-focused so as not to cry in the exam room. Think about this happening with your clinician. Does your clinician stop their current talk track to ask you how you're feeling, or if you any clarification? Do they keep talking as if they don't see you on the brink of tears? Some parts of the healthcare journey are terrifying. Although you have a responsibility as a patient to learn how to express your emotions verbally to your provider, an emotionally intelligent provider will recognize something is wrong and give you an opening to talk instead of acting like everything is okay.

Nurturing a Strong Relationship of Trust

Without trust, you don't have anything substantial. When patients trust their clinical care team, they trust that the team has their best interest in mind and can provide adequate medical care. Trust allows patients to be vulnerable about their feelings and have an open dialogue about the quality of care they receive, what needs to improve, and so much more.

Would you let someone you don't trust house-sit for you while you're out of town? So why should you be willing to keep clinical care team members around to support your healthcare journey whose support is, at best, worthy of a side-eye? Newsflash — you shouldn't. Think about what it takes to say that you trust someone personally. It takes repeating behavior over and over again that is acceptable over time.

Take these steps to nurture the strong relationship you've built with your clinician and your clinical care team:

- **Continue to be prepared to meet with your team:** Coming to your doctor's appointment ready to review new symptoms, give feedback about recent treatment options, and get down to business shows that you value their time.

REMEMBER

Dialogue about healthcare is a two-sided coin. You can build a strong relationship of trust by going to your doctor's appointments, and being very succinct in your communication.

- **Remain actively involved in your care:** You should allow your care team the space to explain their approach, give you their opinion based on their clinical expertise, and present all relevant facts regarding a potential treatment plan. It's important to note that your clinician and clinical team should empower you in a comfortable, trusting relationship to push back and ask questions.

  You show trust when you give your providers the space to present their findings. When your providers create a safe space for you to ask questions or challenge what they say, they show that they trust you and respect your position as the patient.

- **Prioritize honesty during communication:** When you trust someone, you're honest with them. Continuing to have a solid, trusting relationship with your clinical care team means being honest. That means being entirely upfront about your opinion of a treatment option, the medications, your ability to afford medication or other proposed treatment options, and more. Have you ever heard the expression that secrets keep you sick? Secrets can keep you sick, especially when you keep them from your healthcare provider.

REMEMBER

Honesty needs to be present on both sides. You must be honest with your clinician about your feelings and circumstances; however, your clinician must also be honest with you. This means owning up to mistakes when they are made and consciously working to regain any trust that's been lost.

Establishing a Culture of Collaborative Decision-Making

As the patient, you should always be at the center of your care. You should know what options are available, the pros and cons, the treatment plans proposed to help you get from point A to point B, how much they cost, how equitable they are to your situation, and any other relevant information.

To be an informed, empowered patient, you must be part of a healthcare team that prioritizes collaborative decision-making. This means that in your position as the ultimate final say on the team, you can brainstorm options, collect information, and put together the best care plan. This is done in conjunction with the team that has rallied around you. You have the same goal — to get you the best clinical outcomes possible.

REMEMBER

Your position of authority in your care it not diminished by engaging your team in the process, intentionally trying to understand their perspectives, and doing what's right for you based on the information presented.

To foster this culture, you can say things like the following:

It's a priority for me to learn to manage my chronic health condition with lifestyle changes. However, I appreciate your input about the importance of managing this condition with medication as well. The last medication we tried gave me side-effects I'm not comfortable with. Do you have information or perspective on an alternative medication to consider? Also, to support my lifestyle change management goal, who else should we consult with?

With this response, you:

- Clearly outlined your priorities
- Acknowledged the provider's input about the importance of using a medication with lifestyle changes
- Provided feedback about your experience with the last medication
- Expressed openness to continuing the conversation of finding a better medication
- Asked your team's input on finding an additional resource that can help you with your lifestyle changes

You covered a lot of ground in two or three sentences! I say that's worthy of a little happy dance!

IN THIS CHAPTER

» Speaking directly about a subject

» Clarifying confusing conversations

» Speaking confidently and respectfully

» Asking the right questions

Chapter 6
Guiding Your Healthcare Conversations

To make it through the healthcare system with your sanity and to get the results to you are looking for, you need to talk to people — specifically to your healthcare team. By "talking," I don't mean just asking about the weather and other conversational pleasantries, I mean you must know how to *communicate*. Many well-intentioned patients believe that the best way to survive the healthcare system is to not create a "fuss," which they think means not doing too much talking or double-checking because they don't want to come across overbearing.

This chapter breaks down everything you need to know about communicating effectively with your care team to feel empowered, self-assured, and in control regarding conversations about your health. Get ready to watch your health conversations go from passive and vague to productive, meaningful, and clear in no time!

Fine-Tuning Your Direct Conversation Skills

The best communication is clear, calm, focused, and assertive in real time. The following tips go a long way to helping you be direct and clear when communicating with your care team:

- **Speak confidently:** The reason you are having this conversation is to gain a better understanding of the factors related to your healthcare journey. It's important to be very clear on this mental framing. You are in the driver's seat of your own health. Yes, clinical decision making is a collaborative art; however, the final say is yours. Remind herself that you don't need validation or reaffirmation of your position to make important decisions. It's your health. Use "I" statements, ask to stop conversations when you don't understand what's being said, and don't shy away from sharing information about how you feel.
- **Be specific when providing details about your concerns and symptoms:** Your care team needs to understand what is bothering you, how you respond to certain treatments, and other important factors. Learn to communicate about your symptoms by letting your clinician know what the discomfort feels like, when you experience it, how long you experience it, on what part of your body your experience it, if the discomfort or pain stays in one place or if it radiates or moves to other places, and more. Consider sharing details about what makes your symptoms better, what makes your symptoms worse, how frequently you experience symptoms, how long they go away before they come back, and other more specific information that helps guide clinical decision making on their end.
- **Keep your emotions in check:** This is essential to the way that you are perceived and ultimately to the outcomes you receive. To get your emotions in check, start learning how to recognize how you're feeling and why you're feeling it. It's understandable to be upset, overwhelmed, angry, or frustrated with your experience with the healthcare system. Those feelings are valid and do not have to go away; however, you can communicate those feelings with composure. Being composed doesn't mean that you can't cry, or

have a few moments of overwhelm. However, composure means not allowing those emotions to cloud your analytical and strategic analyses. Learn to feel your emotions, recognize them, validate them, and then put them in their place so that you can make the best decision possible.

TIP

When or if you find yourself being emotionally overwhelmed, it is okay to tell the people you're speaking to that you need a few moments to collect yourself. Do not feel pressured to make difficult decisions while you are feeling emotional or overwhelmed. Getting your emotions in check does not mean acting like a robot. You are *allowed* to feel all your emotions, but it is your responsibility to make sure they don't cloud your decision-making capabilities.

- **Prioritize being organized:** Get key information and points on paper or in a format that you can reference quickly and easily.

  By being organized you will have a clear view of all of the factors and can keep your focus during challenging conversations.

- **Be mindful of body language:** If you know you wear your emotions on your sleeve, or better yet your forehead and your face, try to be mindful of that in difficult conversations. The subliminal cues and messages that you give off have a lot to do with the way you are perceived. Being mindful of your body language can contribute to the confidence you exude.

TIP

Take deep breaths to recenter if you become overwhelmed. Avoid negative body language like crossing your arms, rolling your eyes, and other nonverbal cues, when possible.

- **Use assertive language that is strong but respectful:** Being respectful does not mean being docile. If you have a strong position or opinion about something, it's your right and responsibility to make sure that you convey your feelings. First, start by identifying the issue you want to address and then taking a solution-oriented approach to working through it. Use "I" statements and avoid "you" statements. You can say things such as, "I feel that." or "I need." Make sure you provide details and facts to support your "I" statements. You don't have to make yourself small to be respectful.

REMEMBER

Being respectful doesn't mean that you have to be happy and pleasant about navigating the healthcare system. Navigating it is hard and there will be days that you don't feel well. You might feel frustrated, scared, skeptical, and just downright angry. Being respectful also doesn't mean that you have to agree with your healthcare professionals. You can respectfully disagree and do so firmly without engaging in behaviors that make the other parties feel unsafe, demeaned, or insignificant.

Probing for clarity

Conversations in the healthcare setting can often lack clarity, mutual understanding, and be just downright confusing. The important point to remember is that when you are in a confusing conversation, you need to probe for clarity in order to get the information you need.

Questions can range from things like just asking a provider to explain more about a treatment or which specialists you schedule for. If you're having a hard time understanding what is being related to you verbally, you can always ask for visual aids, diagrams, pictures, and other visual aids that will help you understand the process. This is not an uncommon ask and many healthcare professionals are able and equipped to provide such aids (see Figure 6-1).

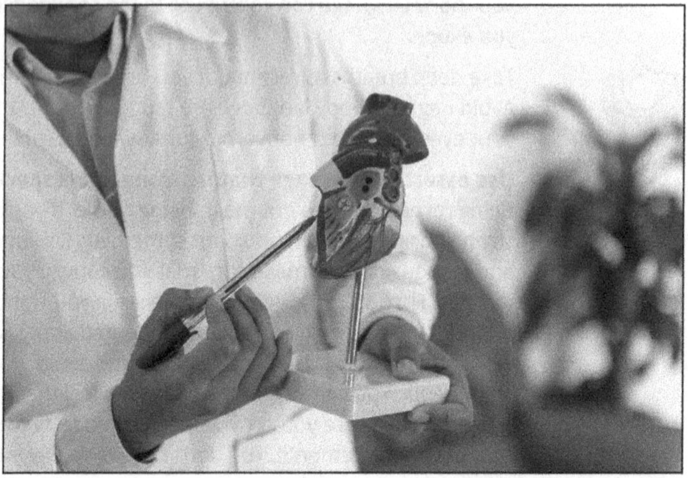

Gerardo Huitrón/Getty Images

FIGURE 6-1: From brochures to 3D models, visual aids can help clarify otherwise confusing concepts.

REMEMBER

There's no shame in letting the person you're speaking with know that you are confused. Repeat back to them what you've heard, what you understand, and what you don't. This allows your care team to better understand what you need from them.

Active listening means listening with the intention to understand, giving the person who's speaking your full attention, and placing an emphasis on comprehension. This is more than just passively hearing the words that are coming out of their mouth. If you are actively listening to what your provider is saying and you still don't understand, that is the moment in which you need to ask them to pause or slow down, let them know that you're confused, explain to them what you do understand, and give them an overview of what you don't.

Identifying what's confusing

When you are attempting to unravel a very confusing conversation, it's important to first pinpoint what part of the conversation is unclear to you. It may sound silly, but it is important to get to the bottom of what is confusing you.

In order for you to help the members of your care team help you understand what's going on, you need to tell them what you don't understand. If you're sitting down with your care team and they are explaining to you the process of how they are going to rule out different conditions you might have and you become confused about what type of tests you need, that is what you need to relate to your care team.

TIP

To get to the bottom of your feelings about what's confusing you about a dialogue, make a mental checklist, or even a physical checklist, of what you *do* understand. Sometimes reading back or relaying what you understand to your provider helps elucidate what you don't understand.

Once you've identified the parts of the dialogue that were confusing, you should start asking very targeted, specific questions. The next section talks more about asking good questions.

Asking the "Right" Questions

In many ways, the concept of what is "right" and what is "wrong" can seem vague and ambiguous. What is "right" or appropriate in one situation can be viewed as "wrong" or inconsiderate in others. So why is it so important to ask the "right" questions? What even is the "right" question? You learn more about that shortly, but let's first consider why it's important to ask the right questions.

When you ask the right questions, you find yourself in a position where you have the information you need, or are beginning to gather the information you need, so that you can make informed decisions about your care — such as how your condition is responding to a treatment, the side-effects of a medication you have to take, or other questions pertaining to your health. As you've learned, being equipped with relevant information about your health positions you to make the best decisions.

What makes a question "right"

Boiling it down, a question that is right is a question whose answer provides the essential information you need to make decisions about your health that align with your values and needs. That's it!

A question that is right for you may not be right for someone else. Many patients hyper-fixate on the idea of what is a correct or incorrect question to ask. The answer is — as you've probably already learned — there are no incorrect questions. There may be an appropriate time and person to ask certain questions to get the best response, but if you have questions at any point, ask!

Taking personal variability out of the equation, some questions are better than others. The best questions are specific, concise, clear, simple, and open-ended. Consider the following scenario:

Maxine needs to start taking a medication for a chronic condition. She wants to know how much the generic version of the medication costs. The right questions in that moment to ask might be, "Does this medication have a generic version"? and "How much is the generic version?"

Open-ended questions are always better too. You want to makes sure that the information relayed to you in response is helpful. So instead of asking your clinician, "Is this surgery necessary?," ask "Why are you recommending this surgery, what are the possible outcomes, and are there any non-surgical alternatives available to me that might achieve the same result?"

Their response will move from a "yes" or "no" to a more in-depth dialogue that will provide the answers you need to make an informed decision.

TIP

If you have a question that your care team cannot answer, ask them if there is a specific department or point of contact you should reach out to get your answer. You can say something like, "Thanks for answering my question. Can you connect me with the department that handles [*insert topic here*] so that I can ask a few more specific questions?"

The impact of strategic questioning on problem solving

Crafting questions whose answers provide crucial information to make the best health decisions for you empowers you to solve the problem. Strategic questioning can be your superpower and can significantly enhance your ability to solve problems in healthcare interactions.

Not only do you shift the complexity of the dialogue from potentially flat "yes" or "no" answers, but you can also begin to open the door to deeper conversations, detailed information, and better understanding about issues that affect your health concerns and treatment plans. This also allows you to map out the questions you need to ask to get specific information about your condition or plan of treatment that you did not have before.

Formulating effective questions

The ability to formulate specific and effective questions about your healthcare journey is a skill that you can develop over time. It is, as I've said, a mindset shift. Taking some time before your appointment to think about the reason you're having the appointment, what you would like to be reviewed during that appointment with big concerns or questions you have about that appointment, and what information you need from your provider is very important.

Starting by understanding the goal of the appointment is key. The questions you ask your clinician during a postoperative appointment after surgery will be different than the ones you ask them during a wellness visit. It's important to remember that any question that is relevant to you at that time is the right question to ask. It's also important to be mindful of why you're meeting and who you're meeting with. For example, if you have very specific, in-depth questions about your gut health, it might be best to direct those questions to the gastroenterologist you're working with, as opposed to a clinician from another specialty.

As mentioned, the best questions are specific, clear, open-ended, and concise. Here are examples of these characteristics:

- **Specific questions:** Questions about a particular topic.

  Good example: "What do the results of my genetic testing tell you about my future risk of cancer?"

  Example that needs work: "Am I going to get cancer?"

- **Clear questions:** Direct with simple, clear language, and no rambling. They are easily understood.

  Good example: "I don't think I can afford my medication this month. What programs are available to me to help cover the cost?"

  Example that needs work: "I'm having trouble with my meds. Can you help?"

- **Concise questions:** Questions that are to the point.

  Good example: "What side effects to this treatment do I need to be aware of?"

  Example that needs work: "Can you explain all the possible ways someone might experience a reaction to this treatment, including presentation between men and women, symptoms, mortality rates, and so on?"

TIP

As you can create your list of questions, consider asking someone close to your healthcare journey, such as a significant other or a friend, to help you. Loved ones may be able to highlight observations that you made and encourage you to add them to the list of questions to share with your clinician.

Speaking Up with Confidence

The idea of having to speak up for your health needs might scare some people. When you tell your clinician and your clinical team what's wrong with you, they're supposed to know what test to perform, what medications to administer, which treatment plans to follow, and how to meet your health needs, right? That's not completely accurate. Your health and wellness is not all clinical. There are other aspects of your health, like your emotional well-being, that can drastically affect your quality of life.

Considerations like social support, fitness programs, mental health status, and other aspects that don't fit cleanly into the idea of clinical care contribute to a holistic health approach. These considerations are often unknown to your care team — that is, until you tell them.

Learning to drive the conversation

Keep these points on mind as you work on speaking up confidently about your healthcare journey:

- **There is no shame in advocating for yourself:** Everyone involved in your care has a vested interest in making sure that you receive the best outcomes possible and can enjoy the quality of life that aligns with your values, goals, and beliefs. If you're not comfortable with a proposed medical treatment, say so. If you don't like the way you're being spoken to by a healthcare professional, say something. There are very few things in life that are customized specifically for you. Thankfully, your healthcare is one of them.
- **Learn as much about your health conditions as possible:** You don't have to go to medical school and study every clinical nuance of your condition. However, the more you know and the more you learn about conditions, processes, treatments, and medications that affect you, the more comfortable you will be having a conversation about them.
- **Make it a rule that every time you don't understand something presented to you, you ask a question:** Whether you ask the question during that appointment, write it down for next time, or do research to answer that question later, making a commitment to yourself empowers you to confidently assert your opinions, values, and expectations as they become relevant.

» **Use "I" statements when communicating about your needs or concerns:** Saying things like I want, I feel, or I need places the ownership on whatever comes next in that sentence to you. Practice speaking in an authoritative manner that is not confrontational or rude.

REMEMBER

You have every right to be involved in your healthcare. You don't owe anyone the keys to drive your care in whatever direction they see fit.

Conquering the fear of being an "annoying patient"

For years, while I worked alongside patients to help them find their voices and hold conversations about their care, I heard the same constant fear rear its ugly head — "I don't want my doctor to think I'm *annoying.*"

Many patients worry that every time they ask a question about their care, ask their provider to repeat something, or disagree with their provider, their provider was thinking about marking their file with a giant A for "annoying."

Jokes aside, let's take a minute to unpack what it means to be "annoying." In the context that some patients think about being annoying, this might mean:

» Asking a lot of questions

» Reading everything before it's signed

» Holding providers accountable by asking follow-up questions

» Seeking second opinions

These aren't the actions of an annoying patient — they are the actions of a patient advocating for themself. When you see them written out this way, I hope you'll agree that it's difficult to categorize those behaviors as annoying. As long as you maintain respect and keep your emotions in check, these are exactly the kinds of questions you should be asking. If your care team disagrees, it might be time to get a new care team.

3

Embracing Your Role as Your Health's Best Advocate

IN THIS PART . . .

Becoming a knowledgeable self-advocate on your own healthcare journey

Effectively advocating for your own health with the best resources and knowledge

Measuring the impact and effectiveness of your self-advocacy

Building your all-star care team, defining care objectives, and cultivating collaborative decision-making

IN THIS CHAPTER

» **Understanding how to productively use your emotions in self-advocacy**

» **Knowing how to check your provider's understanding of what you understand**

» **Cultivating self-awareness to your benefit**

» **Staying organized and other ways to effectively advocate for your own health**

Chapter 7
Self-Advocacy Techniques to Champion Your Health

Understanding how the healthcare system works, your place as a patient in it, and the tools available to pay for your care, protect your rights, and build a strong working relationship with your care team is just the beginning.

Being your best advocate for your healthcare also requires you to be in tune with your feelings and to be able to communicate them. In this chapter, I help you begin your self-advocacy journey. You discover how to double-check that your provider's understanding is aligned with yours by using the teach-back method, and you find out how to communicate your goals about your health to your providers. Lastly, this chapter includes tips and tricks for successfully advocating for yourself.

Getting to the Core of Your Feelings About Your Health

Realizing that you're not happy with the experience you're having with your clinician or the healthcare system, in general, is often the epiphany that you need to achieve a better outcome. Having this epiphany is an excellent step in the right direction! Getting a better healthcare experience might mean hiring a private patient advocate to work alongside you or simply having realignment conversations with your clinical team. In either case, feeling, recognizing, and understanding your frustration means that you're paying attention to what's going on, recognize there's a disconnect, and need something to change.

The relationship between your health, your emotions, and every other decision you make regarding your healthcare are interconnected. To advocate for yourself effectively, you must be in tune with and honor your emotions.

Setting some ground rules for embracing your emotions

One of the most incredible superpowers you have as a patient advocating for your health is your intuition and personal relationship with your feelings. Think about this: No one else has lived in your body and experienced what you are currently experiencing the way you're experiencing it now. You know how your body feels when you're overworked and burning out or when an ache or pain is unusual.

Emotions are valid, and they are important. The frustrations that you feel about your health, the treatment you're receiving, or the support that you are experiencing are valid. The way that you perceive and respond to concerns about your health, how you interact with your care team, and whether you understand your treatment options are all influenced by your emotions. Consider these two points:

- **On the plus side:** There's nothing wrong with having emotions, and when channeled correctly, they can be powerful allies that guide you to the outcomes you're looking for. Emotions are not bad; in fact, they can motivate you to take action.

» **On the flip side:** Even though acknowledging and respecting your emotions is important, you must still make logical, informed decisions that best fit your values and needs. It's important to understand that your feelings and emotions about your health have an impact on your decisions.

WARNING

If you don't take time to understand *why* you feel the way you feel, your judgment can be clouded when making decisions. You might otherwise make impulsive choices that don't align with your best interest in the long run.

So, how do you strike the perfect balance? How do you make decisions that positively acknowledge your emotions but are still informed, analytical, and fact-based? The tips and tricks that you discover throughout this book can help you process your emotions, especially when navigating illness.

Here are other ideas for establishing ground rules for accessing your feelings and emotions:

» **Invest in therapy or counseling:** This way, you can regularly communicate with a provider you trust about your emotions and work on processing them in a way that's helpful to you. As much as they wish they were, healthcare providers are not mind readers and they might have trouble understanding your needs or feelings about your health if you don't tell them.

» **Ask questions about the best ways to communicate respectfully and competently about your emotions:** Doing so will help your providers understand your situation and any mitigating factors better.

Grappling with emotions in a real-life situation

In any situation where you are the patient, you encounter two critical components of self-advocacy. They are

» **Accepting responsibility:** You are responsible for your health journey and mindset as a patient. In this role you must embrace your emotions, use the correct resources, and continuously make decisions that align with your individual values, health goals, and needs.

» **Addressing a non-optimal healthcare situation:** Understanding your emotions offers you the ability to recognize that something isn't right with the current state of your healthcare situation.

TIP

JAMIE'S HEALTHCARE JOURNEY

To illustrate the components of patient self-advocacy, this real-world example (names changed, of course) shows the steps that one patient took to successfully accept responsibility and address what he viewed as a non-optimal healthcare situation.

Jamie's first attempt to address his frustrating healthcare situation. Jamie sustained an injury at work that significantly affected his ability to walk without a mobility assistant, like a wheelchair or a *rollator* (a wheeled, rolling walker). Over several months, he struggled to understand that he might not ever walk without a mobility assistant again. Frustrated, overwhelmed, and a little bit scared, Jamie spent several months getting second, third, and fourth opinions from different doctors, hoping that someone would tell him that he'd be able to walk again without assistance.

Despite seeing numerous doctors, Jamie's prognosis didn't change, and he became increasingly discouraged and angry. At that point in his care, Jamie decided that he needed to work with a professional patient advocate to continue identifying doctors around the country who could give him the answer he was looking for.

Jamie considers for his core emotions by asking himself how he feels about his health, followed by several "why" questions.

Jamie wrote down how he felt about his health and his experience with his clinical team. He wrote about being frustrated and overwhelmed and then asked himself why. He wrote that his doctors kept telling him that he would not be able to walk normally anymore after his accident, and that made him angry. He then asked himself why this information made him angry. Is he angry

- Because the doctors weren't listening to him?
- Because he doubted the doctors' clinical expertise and felt that another doctor would give him a more thorough examination?

- That the doctors were not presenting him with sufficient treatment options?

Jamie determined that he's angry because he felt like his life would be completely different. Again, asked himself why and found that he

- Didn't know how to do the personal activities he likes doing with a mobility aid.
- Won't be able to live and enjoy activities on his own the way he always has.

The answer to this second why question was an important revelation for Jamie and helped him assign a healthcare goal that addressed this situation (because living independently with a condition that affects your mobility may be entirely possible). The additional worry impacted how he felt about his health and, ultimately, his expectations of his care.

Continuous improvement and problem-solving processes commonly use an iterative reasoning technique — called the *five whys* — to identify the root cause of an issue. The method, created by Sakichi Toyoda and made part of the Toyota Production System, prompts an individual trying to solve the problem to define the problem and ask themselves why it's happening five times, where the next "why?" is in response of the previous question's "why."

To use this why technique in a patient self-advocacy situation, don't limit the number of why questions to five. Some problems may call for further deduction. My rule is to ask "why" until you can't answer why anymore.

Jamie used his new-found core of feelings to streamline and redefine his goals for his healthcare. Having uncovered a new core feeling about his health and current situation, he identified the correlation between his feelings about his current situation, which was relatively negative. Knowing that he didn't want to lose his independence helped him create goals and work with his providers to gain resources to aid his accessibility.

Jamie checked his understanding of his core feelings with a positive hypothetical scenario. He wanted to know whether he had

(continued)

(continued)

reached his core feelings about his health, so he checked his understanding with a scenario. He imagined himself getting in and out of his home easily to go to the farmers market around the corner from his house or taking his family on a road trip. He asked himself how he would feel about his health if this were his reality? If Jamie finds that he would be happy, then he's gotten to one of the cores of his feelings about his health. If he finds that he is still not satisfied, he should ask himself why and continue digging.

There may be many core feelings to uncover about your health that may evolve over time — and that's okay. "Gut check" your feelings using the whys tool as often as you need to and establish a relationship with a mental health provider or therapist to help guide you along your journey of self-discovery.

Jamie shared his new health goals with this clinical team and managed the expectations of his care to meet them. How did all of this help Jamie in his interactions with his clinical care team, his doctors, and the healthcare system in general? Well, now Jamie knows more about himself — he identified a priority regarding his quality of life. He can now work with his providers to set goals and achieve those goals actively.

Jamie may decide to abandon the process of getting other opinions about his injury — or maybe he won't. He can continue to advocate for the presentation of other treatment plan options with his doctors.

The exercise about Jamie is not meant to broad-stroke the emotional and physiological complex thought and healing process that comes with an individual experiencing a significant change to their state of being following an injury but present as an additional tool in your arsenal to help you understand why you feel the way you think about your health.

Now it's your turn! Grab a sheet of paper, a journal, or even the blank space on this page and reflect on your emotions about your health over the past couple days:

» Can you think of a few ways those emotions have influenced the decisions you've made about your health in the past?

- Do you feel that you have access to a safe space to further unpack your emotions?
- Have you been able to effectively communicate your emotions to your clinical care team?

Write down the name of the emotion you have been feeling and start asking your "why" questions. This exercise is an important step in the right direction on the journey of confidently advocating for your health and your well-being as a patient.

The better we get to know ourselves, the way we feel, and why we feel that way, the better we are able to communicate what is important to us, what we need to be successful, and why we would like them to engage with us the way that we're asking them to.

Using the Teach-Back Method with Your Providers

Suppose that you're feeling stressed about some new symptoms you're having and have waited months for an appointment with your clinician. The day finally comes for your appointment, and you are sitting in the examination room waiting for your clinician to return after reviewing the imaging and the lab work that they ask you to complete prior to the visit. Here's what happens next:

1. The clinician finally appears in the exam room doorway and begins flying through the talking points of your appointment. They are in and out the door in less than 20 minutes.
2. At the end of your appointment, you're standing in the lobby of your doctor's office, holding an after-visit summary. You don't quite understanding what was said, what you're supposed to do, and why your clinician made the decisions they made to start you on this new medication that you've never heard of.
3. This whirlwind cycle continues when you proceed to follow your doctor's orders to the best of your ability. You come back in a later appointment to report that you're still not feeling well, and even feeling worse.

HEALTHCARE SYSTEMS IN CRISIS

Clinical teams are understaffed, nurses are overworked, doctors are burnt out, and it may seem that there's no end in sight to the damage this does to patient care. Clinical teams and healthcare leaders are doing the best they can to provide top-quality care to patients amid all of the systemic and administrative barriers they are faced with. As a patient, it's okay to have empathy for those who are working tirelessly to provide good quality patient care in a broken system. However, it's also okay to feel that the quality of your care should not be affected by their difficulties. Yes, you can empathize with the clinician who has to see scheduled patients every 20 minutes, but you also want to make sure that that your 20-minute interaction with that clinician is meaningful and that you feel supported, understand the facts of your care, and can make informed decisions about your health.

Does this scenario sound familiar? Although patients enjoy the benefits of biomedical innovations, advanced research, and advanced treatment options, the healthcare system is far from perfect. For one, it's often too understaffed (or undertrained) to provide sufficient individual attention and care. So, what do you do in the moment when your clinical team is barreling information at you at 100 miles per hour and you're struggling to understand them correctly?

An extremely effective strategy for ensuring that you understand and have mutual agreement about the information presented and the next steps proposed is called the *teach-back method.*

Confirming what you understand

Many clinicians actually learn to use the teach-back method to ensure that their patient understands the information they presented to them, but it's not a bad idea to get in the habit of learning the method yourself and using it on your care team, if in the event they do not check for your understanding. The technique involves you, the patient, repeating the information your clinical team has relayed to you back to them in your own words.

By doing this, you begin the process of confirming that you understand what your provider is telling you and that there is clear communication. This method isn't intended to be a tool to quiz you on how much you remember and it's okay if you don't remember everything.

If you don't remember everything, or you remember something differently than your provider explained it, your clinical team now has the opportunity to clarify what they meant or give you additional information to fill in your knowledge gaps.

By the end of this exercise, everyone should be on the same page about the information that was presented, the treatments that were discussed, the findings of any tests that were performed, your health goals, and any next steps. There is also an added benefit for you. When you absorb information and speak it back — or teach it back — to someone else, you are much more likely to understand and remember it.

Learning the teach-back method

Follow these steps to put the teach-back method to use from the patient perspective:

1. **Pay close attention to what you're hearing while you're communicating with your clinical care team members.**

   You have to listen in order to understand. When your provider is explaining the findings of any test they perform, more information about your condition, proposed treatment plans, or medicine, like the introduction of a new drug, listen carefully. Your goal is to understand what is being said so that you can repeat the information later.

   TIP It's helpful to jot down a few notes in a notebook or record your provider's explanation with their permission. It's okay to ask them to slow down or to repeat something.

2. **Repeat what you've heard to your clinical care team member.**

   Focus on summarizing what you've heard in Step 1. The key is to summarize the information in your own words. Don't spend time trying to repeat information verbatim, but repeat it back as if you were speaking informally to a friend, colleague, or someone you trust. You could say things like, "What I heard you say is that I should take the antibiotic twice a day for ten days and then schedule a follow-up appointment if I still feel poorly. Is that correct?"

REMEMBER

Repeating what you hear and then asking for confirmation allows your provider to further clarify their instructions or help you correct your understanding.

3. **Ask your clinical care team member for clarification of any items that you either forgot or aren't sure that you fully understand.**

   After you summarize (Step 2), your clinical care team member may indicate that your summary is not exactly what they meant. Make note of the things that weren't quite clear to you and ask for clarification. You might say something like, "Could you explain what you mean by 'checking my levels'?" Remember — this is your opportunity to ask questions!

   TIP

   Don't worry if you forget to ask a question during your appointment. Add a reminder in your phone and assign a date and a time to it.

   If phone reminders are not your thing, write down your question on a sheet of paper by your phone, or your computer, or another dedicated place where you sit down to contact your doctor's office.

4. **Confirm your provider's understanding of your understanding.**

   To wrap up the process, once you've had the opportunity to repeat information back in your own words and work through any corrections with your provider, confirm with your provider that they understand what you've taken from the conversation. You could say something like, "That's what I've taken from our conversation. Do you feel like we're on the same page?"

   Asking this question prompts your provider to make an assessment of their perception of your understanding. If they feel like you weren't quite catching the critical elements of the information they've shared with you, they have another opportunity to rectify that.

Consider these points regarding the purpose and benefits of using the teach-back method:

- **Shared understanding:** By using the method, you build a shared understanding of your healthcare issues and action points.

» **Patient-centered interaction:** No one benefits from a relationship where you, as the patient, take marching orders from your clinical team without understanding why you're being asked to do. Your interactions with your clinical team should enhance your understanding of the complexities of your healthcare.
» **Assurance of active participation:** By initiating the process, you can almost ensure your active participation in every conversation and decision about your health.

Sharing Your Health Goals with Your Providers

When planning for any success, it's common to think of the phrase "begin with the end in mind." This thought process can be helpful because it allows you to disregard the uncertainty and cloudiness of your current situation and envision the end goal. Think about trail hiking on a very foggy, gray day and seeing a red flag far off in the distance, which signifies the end of the trail. In that moment you probably don't know what the first five feet of terrain looks like in front of you because of all the fog, but you have a general idea of the direction that you want to go and when you're going to stop hiking.

This is what managing a health condition can feel like. Partnering with your clinical care team, it's extremely important to set clear, achievable health goals that can help positively influence your health outcomes. But how do you set them? How do you know if they're achievable? Can your goals change? You explore these questions in this section.

Making sure your goals are SMART

When setting any kind of goal, health related or not, a common helpful framework to utilize is the SMART approach. This approach, first popularized by George T. Doran, is used in corporate and professional settings to create a systematic framework for describing the components of a goal, denoted by the acronym SMART (specific, measurable, achievable, relevant, and time-bound).

I use SMART goals to create a sense of structure to goal-setting because it forces me to break large, sometimes ambiguous, goals into something more bite sized and actionable.

A healthcare-related example of this is wanting to manage your diabetes better. This is a complicated goal because the management of diabetes is multifaceted, and it requires action and attention in multiple areas to work well. The term "better" is also subjective.

Managing diabetes "better" for Cassandra, who is struggling to moderate her refined sugar intake, could look completely different than for Kitty, who is trying to be more active. By creating SMART goals, Cassandra and Kitty can both clearly define what they need to do, how to measure it, an achievable way to meet the goals, how relevant they are to their current state, and the time in which they will complete the goals.

Consider Cassandra's health goal of wanting to better manage her diabetes. Her general goal might be, "I want to manage my diabetes better." But a SMART goal like this one would be much more helpful:

"By the end of the month, I will be more mindful of the number of sodas I drink by tracking my intake in my food journal. Over the course of the month, I'll reduce the number of sodas I drink from 10 to 7 to support my goal of managing my diabetes and improving my health."

Cassandra's goal is now SMART:

- **Specific,** because it identifies what she will reduce. In this example, she is reducing the number of sodas she is consuming.

  TIP

  When you make health goals specific, you introduce a level of accountability by making multiple aspects of that goal more clear. When things are clear you know why they're important, when they should be done, how you're going to do them, and how you're going to measure them.

- **Measurable,** because she is tracking it in her food journal.
- **Achievable,** because she is reducing her soda intake by three sodas by the end of the month. It's important to be

realistic in setting goals so that you can make tangible progress and not become frustrated by unrealistic goals.

- **Relevant,** because the action (reducing the amount of soda she drinks) has a direct impact on her diabetes by affecting the amount of sugar she consumes.
- **Time-bound,** because it has a deadline. She's giving herself a month to make the reduction. Setting deadlines fosters accountability because the expectation for completion is not open-ended.

REMEMBER

You can ask your clinical team for help in identifying SMART health goals and in determining which goals will make the most difference to your health. Figuring out how to prioritize goals and how to achieve them can be a collaborative effort with your clinical team, but it's your responsibility to be prepared and open to starting the conversation.

TIP

It's important to document your health goals, on your phone, computer, or on a sheet of paper. Writing goals out helps you clearly articulate what you want to see and helps you remember what you want to communicate to your clinician.

Setting health goals with your care team

Setting goals for your health is one of the most important steps you can take in taking control of your health. This just means taking your SMART goal and drilling down on it to a more micro level.

You can think of the health goal process as a funnel; see Figure 7-1. The top of the funnel, the widest part, is your general goal.

- **Cassandra's general health goal is to manage her diabetes better:** It would appear at the top of the funnel. There isn't much detail to this goal and that's okay, as more specifics are outlined as she moves down the funnel.
- **Cassandra's SMART goal is to reduce her soda intake from ten to seven cans within a month:** In the middle of the funnel is the SMART goal. For Cassandra, this is her goal to reduce her soda intake from ten cans to seven. At the very bottom of the funnel is the collaborative plan with your provider. These are smaller goals that you need to achieve to meet your SMART goal.

» **Cassandra's collaborative action plan with her provider identifies specific ways she can achieve her SMART goal:** For Cassandra, at the bottom of her funnel might be goals like buying a food journal by the end of the week so she can start recording her soda intake, or Cassandra's endocrinologist writing her a referral to a dietician to support her journey.

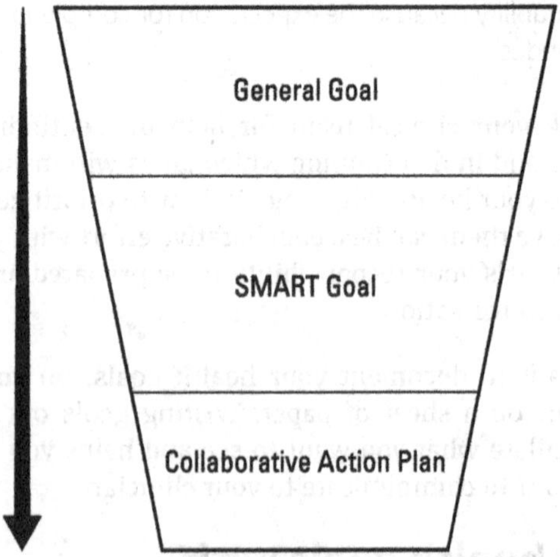

FIGURE 7-1: The process funnel for setting and meeting goals.

Prioritizing your health goals

The next step is the prioritization of your goals with your clinical team. Now that you have an idea of what you want to see done first, you can engage your providers in a conversation of what goals could offer you the most clinical reward first as well. Suppose you injure your knee. Here's what happens next:

» After a knee injury, your goal might be to jump back into your gym routine the way it was before your injury so that you can continue training for your half marathon.

» You communicate to your clinician your goal, but your clinician feels the most clinical benefit is first to prioritize physical therapy specific to your injury.

REMEMBER

Working with your clinical team offers you strategies to put your goals in the right line order, especially if you have a lot of them. Some goals will overlap and other goals can be achieved simultaneously — which is great — so having these conversations with your team can make your goal planning more efficient.

Here's what you know should about health goals:

- Setting health goals is important to self-advocacy.
- Be sure to understand how your health goals align with your feelings about your health.
- Document your health goals.
- There is collaborative benefit in prioritizing goals with your care team.

It's time to start the conversation. Clinical providers like to engage in dialogue about how to problem solve and achieve objectives with you about your health, when prompted.

To start, you could say something like this:

"I've been taking some time to think about what I want from my care and set some goals for myself. A few of the larger goals I have for myself are to [insert broader goals], and I would like your help to turn these goals into ones that are more specific and achievable. What are your suggestions on what we should prioritize first?"

From here, you might find that the conversation evolves naturally. You get into a good groove of brainstorming and the ideas are flowing like the wind. On the other hand, you might get a blank stare from your provider. In either scenario, it's important to make sure you have control of the conversation in a way that is productive and respectful.

Your experience may go either way, so be prepared with appropriate responses by

- **Solidifying the details of your goals:** If you feel the conversation is going well your and brainstorming is evolving, make sure that as you fill out the specifics of your health goals with your provider. It's okay to say something like, "How do I make that goal achievable in three months?" or "How should I measure my improvement?" Once you have all your components accounted for, repeat back the goal in its entirety and make sure it makes sense to both of you.

» **Clarifying your role in setting goals:** If you feel like you are experiencing resistance from your provider such as, feeling rushed to move to the next point or feeling as if your concerns are being dismissed, you could say something like this, "I understand we have a lot to cover during this appointment, and I appreciate your cooperation and having this conversation with me, as it's important for me to set goals for myself about my health. It's important to me to be able to [Insert larger goal], What small steps can I take to get there between now and our next appointment?"

Adjusting and refining your goals

Just like anything else in life, as time passes, things change. Your favorite food in middle school may not be your favorite food now. The amount of sleep you needed ten years ago is probably not the amount of sleep you need now. The same is true for your health goals. Because you change along with the progression of your health journey, your goals will too.

What does this mean for your health goal setting process? It means that the process is never complete. Get comfortable moving through the steps of defining and refining your health goals. If you are managing a long-term condition or a chronic illness, your baseline condition may change with time. Remember, patient self-advocacy is like many other journeys to wellness — the journey doesn't end, it evolves and becomes a process in life that you continue to manage.

The two main steps you need to take when communicating with your clinical team about adjusting your health goals are the following:

1. **Start the conversation by acknowledging the changes in your condition, good or bad.**
2. **Ask your clinician for suggestions on pivoting between goals.**

REMEMBER

The collaboration needed to meet your health goals between you and your provider is a relationship. Healthy relationships require open communication, mutual respect, and empathy. Be sure to respectfully communicate with your care team but don't let them dismiss your observations or concerns. If you experience pushback from your provider, restate your priorities. It's your responsibility to voice your observations and concerns respectfully, and it is also your provider's responsibility to provide you with the tools and clinical expertise to meet them.

IN THIS CHAPTER

» Fostering self-awareness

» Learning to do research with reliable resources

» Recognizing your personal strengths

» Making self-compassion a priority

Chapter 8
Empowering Self-Advocacy Through Knowledge

Achieving the personalized healthcare you desire requires you to commit to lifelong patient self-advocacy. Every healthcare interaction requires you to remain present while understanding available resources and being conscious of your strengths and weaknesses expectations, and remain aware of your expectations for your healthcare.

Whew! That's a lot of responsibility! Don't worry — you don't have to do all of these things overnight (there's no final destination for being a rockstar self-advocate — it's a journey).

In this chapter, I teach you how to step up your self-advocacy game by emphasizing the importance of identifying and utilizing credible sources, broadening your awareness of effective methods to adjust your goals on your health journey as time passes, and doing homework on your strengths and weaknesses as a self-advocate.

Understanding the Impact of Self-Awareness

From an early age, you learn to be observant and respectful of other people's emotions, interact with those around you courteously, and function in society. These skills are critical and can take you a long way (after all, pushing your classmate out of the way to get the last juice box isn't cool). But how much time have you spent learning how to interact with yourself? Are you able to healthily recognize, process, and regulate your emotions? How about your triggers and pet peeves? If you're not quite there yet, that's okay.

Building self-awareness allows you to understand your relationship with your emotions and, ultimately, with yourself. Once you become aware of how you react to certain situations, what your emotions mean, and how to work through them, you become more confident in yourself and in situations where you must advocate for your needs.

By doing this self-discovery work, you set yourself up to be:

- A better decision maker
- More articulate about what works for you and what doesn't
- Able to foster and maintain healthy relationships
- Less stressed
- A happier person

Self-awareness is a form of personal growth and the cornerstone of many other personal growth phenomena, including emotional intelligence. As you begin to learn, you can transform the way you understand and interact with people.

Recognizing your strengths and weaknesses

Nobody is perfect. Even the most poised, put-together individuals have aspects of their personality they want to improve. Even though personal strengths and weaknesses can feel subjective, most people have a general sense of what they are good at and what they need to need to improve upon. Identifying the unique qualities that make you who you are and reflecting on areas to improve can help you on your healthcare journey. If you feel too close to the trees and can't see the forest, ask someone you trust for their opinion.

WARNING

Many say they are okay with constructive criticism — until they receive some. If you are preparing to have an open and honest conversation with someone close to you about their perceptions of your strengths and weaknesses, put yourself in the appropriate frame of mind. The insights you're asking for aren't a personal attack and knowing them can help you improve.

Here are a few ways you can learn about your personal strengths and weaknesses:

- **Think about past experiences and how you have reacted to difficult situations:** Did you find that you are relatively calm under pressure? Do you remember feeling like your head would pop off your body because you were so mad? Think about what parts of those experiences were good or that you were proud of, and opportunities for improvement. Hindsight is always 20/20. It can be helpful to jot down your reflections about a couple of experiences in a journal and make a two-column list of what you did well at and what you felt you could improve upon. You can keep this private.
- **Ask someone you trust how they perceive your strengths and weaknesses:** You can ask them questions about your behavior in various scenarios like "What are some things you think I do well and two things I could improve on when I'm in a situation when I don't feel heard?" or "How do I act when I realize someone is being treated poorly? What could I do better?"

  REMEMBER

  You can't control how someone feels (everyone is responsible for their own emotions), but you are responsible for your actions and should respect people's boundaries.
- **Think about what inspires you and what you struggle to get through:** Chances are, you enjoy doing things that you're good at while you may dread doing things that you are hard for you.

Think about what you love to do and ask yourself why you feel that way. Add these insights to your strengths and weaknesses journaling.

Tools for enhancing self-awareness

You don't have to go to the top of a mountain to find self-awareness. Self-awareness is a journey; luckily, many tools, techniques, and practical strategies can help you dial into your own needs and reactions as you progress on your journey.

Here are some tools and techniques to help enhance your self-awareness journey:

- **Personality assessments** like Myers Briggs Type Indicator (MBTI), the SparkeType test, and the Enneagram test can provide personal insights about your traits, personality framework, and motivations, which can support you on your journey to learn more about yourself.
- **Professional therapy** can provide confidential, personalized insights with a professional to help you understand your motivations.
- **The Wheel of Life exercise** is an activity that helps you visualize what's essential in your life and how all the components balance (see `wheeloflife.io` for more information).

Discerning Information Sources as Friend or Foe

The Internet provides access to an abundance of information and has changed the way that we research and find community (there's a good chance that you're reading this book on an e-reader). With so much information at our fingertips, it can be challenging to decipher which sources offer reputable insights and advice about medicine, disease, wellness strategies, or tips on living a healthier life.

In this section, you learn the importance of distinguishing credible resources from other offerings on the Internet, how to avoid potentially harmful misinformation, and how to present your research about an illness or condition to your clinician.

Recognizing credible information sources

Almost anyone with a solid Internet connection and a working keyboard can provide their personal insights and thoughts about any topic on the Internet. This can be a good thing, such as when you're looking for a great blueberry muffin recipe, but it's a concerning when you are trying to gather information about a health condition. When you're looking for medical information, it's obviously better to hear from an expert, not from anyone off the street.

Consider these tips when assessing the credibility of a health-related resource or website:

- **Look for websites run by medical institutions, government agencies, and nonprofit organizations:** Web addresses that end in .edu, .gov, or .org are more likely to be reputable. Organizations like the National Institutes of Health (see Figure 8-1), the U.S. Center for Medicare and Medicaid, and the U.S. Food and Drug Administration (FDA) all have websites that end in .gov. Academic institutions and universities use .edu, and nonprofits like the American Cancer Society use .org.

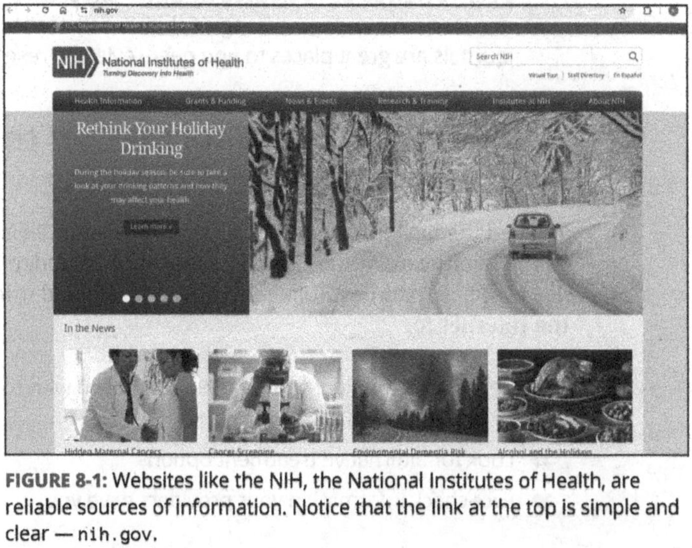

FIGURE 8-1: Websites like the NIH, the National Institutes of Health, are reliable sources of information. Notice that the link at the top is simple and clear — `nih.gov`.

WARNING

Just because you see one of these web address endings doesn't automatically mean that that source is reputable. Be sure to determine who the author of the website is. In everything, use discretion.

- **Verify credentials and qualifications:** Before you read a medical article, search for the credentials of the authors, such as medical training, fellowship completion, association with professional organizations and boards, and so on. Make sure the authors know their stuff!

WARNING

People can be whatever, or whoever, they want on the Internet. Double-check that the article you're reading is written by the person assumed to be the author. Some pesky websites are good at *clickbaiting* and will set you up to believe a falsity. (Clickbait is content on the Internet that' usually sensational or exaggerated so that it encourages people to click on it. It's almost always misleading, and often incorrect.)

- **Determine who funds the website:** If a web page is associated with or paid for by a prominent academic medical center, a large nonprofit organization, or a government agency, it will be noted on the web page. Look out for sites that are funded by random businesses that are trying to sell you something.
- **Make sure that the research studies and articles are peer-reviewed or evaluated by other experts for accuracy:** Pubmed.gov, Google Scholar, and academic journals are great places to find peer-reviewed research.

Using third-party information to enhance your critical thinking

Trusted medical information can empower your decision-making in the healthcare system, but it's essential to understand how to use these sources best. Use reputable and verified information on the Internet to:

- Research a condition you've been diagnosed with to attempt to better understand it.
- Look for alternative treatment options.
- Fact-check information your providers gave you.

Gather your information sources, review them, ask questions, and work with your clinician to determine how it might apply to your case, any viable treatment options, and more. You're showing your clinician that you are interested in your condition and want to be a partner in treating it properly.

Consider using these helpful phrases when presenting information you've gathered about your condition to your clinician:

- "I researched [*insert your condition*] and found that [*insert treatment option*] might help control my symptoms. Can we discuss if this treatment option is right for my situation?"
- "I read on [insert reliable resource here] that lifestyle changes like [*list lifestyle changes*] could complement my current treatment plan. Do you agree? If so, how can we implement them?"
- "I value your clinical expertise and would appreciate your insights on these treatment options I learned after reviewing this research study. What do you think?"
- "I appreciate your guidance as we work to find a diagnosis for my symptoms. I found an article on [*insert source name*] that suggests my symptoms might be caused by [*insert possible diagnoses*]. Have we ruled these out? What are your thoughts?"

TIP

Bring a printed copy of any research studies or articles you want to refer to. This way, your doctors can review them on their own time. Also keep a copy to flip through during your office visit.

Finding a Middle Ground When Reality and Goals Diverge

Sometimes, as patients continue their journey through the healthcare system, they realize that their goals for their healthcare need to align better with their current or future reality. For example, perhaps your initial goal when you started experiencing abdominal pain was to make the abdominal pain go away. Along your health journey, you come to realize that your abdominal pain is part of a chronic condition and may not go away. So your new goal is to manage the pain as best you can.

Being adaptable to the changes of your healthcare story and learning to balance your goals with the reality of your current situation will help you be resilient and stay motivated to continue the journey. Adjusting your health goals as your journey evolves takes strength. You can better meet new goals, define your own happiness, and garner support as your story unfolds.

Prioritizing Self-Compassion

Just because you must adjust your goal doesn't mean you've failed. Practice being kind to yourself, recognize your resilience in setting goals for your help, and work to meet them. It takes immense self-motivation, reflection, and strength to actively manage a condition, navigate a broken healthcare system, gather as much information as possible to make the right decision, and realize that your goals may need to change due to current circumstances. You should not take this lightly.

TIP

Prioritize activities and spend time with people who emotionally support you and help you remain motivated. You've made progress, and no one can take that away!

IN THIS CHAPTER

» **Measuring your self-advocacy efforts**

» **Learning how to receive feedback effectively**

» **Identifying milestones along the way**

Chapter 9 Gauging the Impact of Your Self-Advocacy

So you've realized the importance of championing your own healthcare journey. If you've already invested time into learning how to be the best self-advocate you can be and have begun making changes to the way you prepare for clinical appointments, work with your clinical care team and support system, and care for yourself, congratulations! But how do you know whether your efforts are making a real difference?

In this chapter, you learn practical tips and approachable strategies to evaluate the effectiveness and impact of your self-advocacy. I help you navigate how to quantify your progress, identify areas where you can amplify your voice, as well as facilitate conversations with your clinical care and support teams to measure the success of your efforts.

Measuring Your Efforts

In order to objectively understand how well you are advocating for yourself and how well your efforts are received, you need to evaluate whether your health outcomes align with your expectations and goals.

Measuring the success of your advocacy efforts allows you to hold yourself accountable, refine your strategies, and be able to communicate your wants and needs for improvement or sustain progress to other members of your team.

You want to make sure that the healthcare experience you desire is in alignment with your actual experience. Ask yourself these questions:

- Do I feel heard?
- Are my values being respected?
- Do I feel like I know what's going on with my healthcare?
- Am I confident that I'm communicating effectively and clearly about the expectations I have for each part of my care team?

If you answer no to one or more of these questions, you may need to improve your approach. Think about the "North Star" idea — imagine your best case scenario. For many patients, that means getting all relevant information about multiple aspects of care, being empowered to make informed decisions about their futures, having a clear idea about how much the tests and services cost, and being able to communicate effectively to every member of their team.

Even if you have not achieved every goal in your utopian healthcare ideal, measuring the impact of your efforts allows you to take a step back, appreciate the progress you've made, think about how you are physically and psychologically responding, and ultimately improve the experience.

Getting Feedback Effectively

To measure success, you need to start gathering various types of information in the form of feedback. Feedback is integral to the growth and success of any initiative, program, treatment, or intervention. You need something to evaluate in order to come to conclusions about progress.

So, how do you give it? What do you do when you get it? How do you use it effectively? The following sections dive deeper into considerations about feedback.

Proactively seeking feedback

The right kind of feedback opens doors to insights that you might not have otherwise had. It allows you to see the impact of your advocacy efforts from a different perspective in a more quantitative, unbiased way. In addition, it allows you to communicate with other members of your healthcare team.

There are two types of feedback, self-reflective feedback, and feedback you get from other people (or external feedback). They are both important. Your healthcare journey is about you — point, blank, period. Members of your care team do want to make your experience better. You want to make your experience better because you are directly affected by the complexity and hurdles of a sometimes inefficient, overly complicated system.

In some situations, a patient may be navigating a condition that is not quantitatively, clinically improving. However, after implementing various self-advocacy practices and techniques, they feel like their healthcare actions have improved, because they know how to address certain challenges, they feel that they have been presented with the relevant information, and they feel that their voice is being heard.

Feedback from other people, or external feedback, allows you to hear the perspectives of those close to your care or providing your care. Questions you can ask your care team include:

- Is there anything different I can do to better prepare for my appointments?
- Have I made my health goals and milestones clear?
- Have I worked with you (as my provider or clinical support system) to establish goals that are achievable?

REMEMBER

The decision is ultimately yours regarding what information you want to consider and what information you can respectfully disregard. Try to strike a balance between being sure of yourself and how you feel and valuing the input of other people you trust.

Normalizing the feedback process

Chances are, unless you are dealing with some very opinionated, forward people, you have to ask for feedback. You might have some more assertive personalities in your life who don't mind providing feedback unsolicited. But, generally, you have to ask people to provide their perspective because they don't want to come across as overreaching, hypercritical, or imposing.

To start the conversation, you can open up by staying "Over the past few [days, weeks, months], I've been making an intentional effort to advocate for myself in conversations about my healthcare, and I am preforming a pulse check to see if my efforts have been effective. I would love to get your feedback."

This can break the ice and is a great segue to collect some helpful insights. Be sure that you are clear about the areas you are asking someone to give you feedback on. If you start asking rambling, unfocused questions, you're going to lead people to give you rambling, unfocused answers, or leave them at a point where they don't even know what you want from them.

Depending on who you're talking to, you could ask questions like these:

- "When I'm working with you and you ask me questions about how I feeling or managing my condition, do you feel like I give you clear, specific information about my symptoms, like what makes them better or worse?"
- "At our last appointment, when we discussed starting a new medication, how did you know I fully understood the treatment plan?"

After you ask questions, make an intentional effort to listen to the feedback from a positive, growth mindset. Remind yourself that you are collecting feedback to reach a shared goal. Encourage members of your team to be honest with you and make sure that they understand that you view criticism as constructive.

TIP

As you are gathering crucial information, make sure you are keeping a record of what you heard, your initial thoughts for addressing the feedback, and some steps you can take initially to move in the right direction.

Of course, if you feel as if the criticism or feedback is not constructive and is meant to be malicious or hurtful, you can respectfully disregard those comments. As time goes on, revisit your journal or notes. Make sure to note the date you receive the feedback, from whom you received it, and regarding what specific topic.

Managing the Pitfalls of Collecting Feedback

Receiving feedback about a personal performance or attribute can be difficult. It's not uncommon for people to over-analyze feedback and wonder if it's personal. This is a normal experience of being human. In order to receive feedback with an attitude of openness and curiosity, people must keep their initial personal feelings in check.

There are typical pitfalls that can hinder your ability to receive, comprehend, and utilize feedback. The following sections cover some of these considerations to watch out for.

Hearing only what you want to hear

Otherwise known as *selective hearing*, this can happen when you are having a conversation with someone who is presenting a mixed bag of topics — meaning that they have very positive feedback in some areas, while in others, they note opportunities for improvement. In this scenario, it's human nature to focus on the positive feedback and more or less ignore or forget the other parts.

Of course, you should celebrate positive feedback. However, you're doing yourself a disservice if you ignore any opportunities for improvement. Your healthcare journey is extremely personal, one of the most personal experiences you have. If you make it a priority to build a team of professionals and support partners whose expertise, judgment, and support you trust, you are doing yourself a disservice by not at least considering the feedback they have for you in ways that you can improve.

This is another good reason to take notes on everything. Allow yourself some time to cool down and for the sting of the criticism to die down, then return to your notes. Once you're calmer, you may be able to see this "criticism" as the helpful feedback.

Avoiding feedback

It can be very helpful to get the perspectives of those close to you. Some people avoid collecting feedback because they dread the potential criticism of negative feedback, or they may not understand why it's important.

If you find yourself not wanting to collect feedback from other members of your care team, take a second to pause and ask yourself why that is:

- Do you feel like you're avoiding a negative response?
- Do you feel like your perspective is the only one that you want to consider at this time?
- Do you not know how to collect feedback and want further guidance?
- Is there something else?

You don't have to share this with anyone else. However, giving yourself an opportunity to address why you feel the way you feel helps you plan your next steps forward.

Taking feedback too personally

This can really throw a monkey wrench into your progress. It's helpful to reframe your thinking and understand that the feedback you are receiving is about the processes you manage, the clarity and frequency of the communication you make, and other more tactical aspects of your healthcare journey. It should not be viewed as an attack on your character.

WARNING

People have intuition for a reason, and sometimes, the wrong kinds of people actually do give feedback from a place of judgment or personal critique instead of a place of improvement. If you feel like a professional is making hurtful or inappropriate comments, reach out to resources like the hospital ombudsmen if you are not comfortable addressing them yourself.

Fearing retaliation or scrutiny

Asking members of their care teams about their perceptions keeps some patients from asking questions. Some patients fear that they are asking their care team to grade them on the efforts. They worry about being perceived as skeptical and critical about their the expertise of their care team. They worry that this could possibly lead to strained relationships, reduced quality of care, or even neglect.

Healthcare professionals who perceive a patient's active involvement in their care as being too nosy or over-corrective are not doing their jobs. This is not in the best interest of the patient. If this is your experience, it might be time to find a different care provider.

REMEMBER

You have the fundamental right to understand every aspect of your care, including how it's paid for, what your financial responsibilities are, and your condition, and to be a part of the treatment conversations and plans.

The good news is that most healthcare professionals and care team members welcome and support patient empowerment and self-advocacy. They are more than happy to rally behind patients who want to receive the best medical care possible and want to understand how to work with the professionals on their team in a respectful, collaborative manner, to achieve the best health outcomes.

To squash this fear, let your care team know that you value the collaborative atmosphere you've built with them and that you view feedback as a constructive part of the patient/care provider relationship.

Why timing matters

Determining the best time to have a check-in conversation with your healthcare team can help ensure that it's taken in the way it is intended.

Consider this scenario: You go to your favorite coffee shop to get your usual latte before work. You have always had a great experience with the baristas and enjoy the atmosphere. Today, the shop is very busy. You order your usual latte and wait for it to be prepared. When you get your drink, you realize that it's the wrong size and had too much cinnamon. Moments later, you see one of your favorite servers whizzing by with cups in hand to complete other orders. You decide to let them know that your order was prepared incorrectly. This server, who is usually very patient and accommodating, is very busy today. You sense that your feedback does not land as you intend.

You of course have every right to communicate about the quality of your coffee and provide feedback about your service, but the timing in which you chose to do it, in the middle of the morning rush, affects the reception and may be even your ability to reach a resolution that you are happy with.

Once you're ready to collect feedback from your team, be mindful of how much time you have for the conversation, the craziness of the day, and other factors that can potentially affect the quality of feedback you receive.

If you know that your doctor is running behind, it might be best to initiate a check-in conversation at another appointment when there is more time available to talk. By the same token, plan to have conversations when you do not feel rushed. If you know that you have back-to-back appointments, a soccer game to attend after this appointment, or a meeting to get to, consider this conversation for another day.

Striking the right balance between how frequently you ask for feedback and why you need it is important. You want to have conversations and discussions that are mutually beneficial, that don't overwhelm either party, and that serve a purpose. Consider starting with quarterly or monthly check-ins and then adjusting the frequency to fit the complexity of your healthcare needs, preferences, and other information that is relevant to you.

Seeking professional help when self-advocacy is not enough

Navigating the healthcare system — even despite your best efforts — can be a very difficult task. You might feel like you've done everything right, but you still think that you're not making as much progress as you'd like.

Thankfully, there are professional patient advocates who have extensive training, expertise, and backgrounds who can help you. They have made a professional, personal, and often lifelong commitment to helping patients receive the best quality of care they can. Check out Chapter 19 to learn more about when working with a professional patient advocate, like a board certified patient advocate, independent or private patient advocate makes the most sense, and how to get started.

Realizing that you need help doesn't mean that you're a failure or that you've given up. There's no shame in asking for help. Knowing when to seek help shows that you're strong and savvy. It's what the best leaders do!

Identifying Milestones

Benchmarks and milestones are key ways to measure progress, change, and growth. Being able to establish and recognize milestones allows you to paint a clear picture of your progress, foster motivation, and give you goals to work toward. It's important to set milestones that are personalized to the support your needs and the changes you want to see in your healthcare. They also need to be realistic within a certain time frame.

One patient's self-advocacy milestone might be learning to understand their emotions and successfully communicate concerns about a treatment plan to their care team. Another patient's patient self-advocacy milestone might be making an informed decision about which treatment plan they want to use to manage their condition.

Whatever milestones you choose to guide your progress, give you something to work toward, and celebrate, they need to be yours and yours alone. Learn to work collaboratively with your care team to identify milestones that will be beneficial to multiple parts of your care.

REMEMBER

Your patient's self-advocacy journey is extremely personal and is unlike anyone else's journey because there isn't anyone else like you. Tailor your milestones to your unique healthcare journey. Think about the progress you want to make and what tangible scenarios, conversations, or tasks have to happen.

Achieving milestones and goals allows you to recognize the progress you've made. They should also be reflective of your values, wants, and needs along your healthcare journey. Choose them wisely and don't be afraid to revisit or revise them if they no longer serve you.

Building checklists

Checklists can help you get to the core of what you expect from your healthcare and then you can move further in identifying milestones and goals. You can use this as a self-reflective tool as well. Here are a couple of examples:

- **Communication:** Do you know what's going on with your healthcare? Are you leaving your appointments feeling confused? When you have a question about your healthcare, do you feel like you can ask? Are you experiencing constant miscommunication between your clinical care team, specialist, or support system? Do you feel like your care team's goals are different than yours?

» **Personalization of care:** Do you feel like you are at the center of all your healthcare decisions? Is your treatment custom made for you or does it feel like one-size-fits-all? Does your team ask you questions about how possible treatment plans complement your lifestyle, preferences, and beliefs? Does your care team make you feel strange or unreasonable when advocating for interventions? Do feel safe expressing your individuality and having conversations about how your identity and lifestyle affects your care?

» **Finances and affordability:** Do you understand your financial obligations to your insurance company and healthcare system? Do you know whom to talk to when you receive a bill that is incorrect or incomplete? Do you feel comfortable sharing that you might have additional considerations or are worried that a treatment or medication is too expensive? Are you aware of the financial resources and options you have to ensure that your care is affordable, like payment plans, financial assistance programs, and supplemental insurances? Do you feel like you are receiving different treatment because you have financial limitations?

» **Decision-making as an equal partner:** Do other members of your clinical care and support team value your opinion in conversations about planning your care? Are your preferences being ignored? Are you being consulted about changes to your treatment plans and healthcare steps before they happen? Do you feel like an equal partner along your healthcare journey? Do you feel heard when you speak? Does your care team acknowledge what you say as important? Do you feel empowered to hold members of your care team accountable when the care you receive does not meet your expectations?

» **Respect and comfort:** Are you being treated with dignity? Are members of your team making a conscious effort to ensure that you don't feel dismissed? Do you know what resources are available to address disrespectful or unprofessional behavior? Do you feel like you are being retaliated against or treated differently because you made your expectations of respect and professionalism known? Do you know who to talk to when an issue arises?

As you create your checklist of non-negotiables, add any expectations you have for your care. It will be easier to set milestones and goals that support them. Customize your checklist as much as needed to ensure that it accurately reflects your expectations. Your interactions with your healthcare team are some of the most intimate, serious, and complex interactions you'll have and they can be life or death.

You should expect to receive care that is clinically excellent, meaningful, and adaptive to your needs.

Using technology to track your progress

Once you've identified the milestones you want to meet through the course of your healthcare journey, it's imperative that you record all the steps you've taken to improve your healthcare journey. This could include simply coming prepared to your doctor's appointments with questions, keeping your medication list up to date, and speaking up for yourself.

TIP

Online health management tools, like MyChart, are great tools to have and utilize, especially for communicating to members of your clinical care team. You can schedule appointments, see how many appointments you've attended, message your providers, see how frequently you talk to your providers, access test results and labs, and so much more. See Appendix A for more information about using online health tools.

By becoming familiar with the technological tools at your disposal, you can enhance your patient self-advocacy efforts and have relevant data to look back on and assess how things are going. This allows you to effectively measure the impact of your actions as you continuously improve and refine your approach.

Improving based on feedback

Now that you know the importance of feedback, how to collect it, and how to interpret it in context of your expectations and goals for your healthcare, this section considers what it means to continuously improve your efforts.

The important mindset shift you can make in the evaluation of your efforts is to understand that missteps will happen and you will make mistakes. You may have conversations where the objectives you share are not very clear, or you opt to have a conversation with a member of your team at a difficult time and get the answer you're looking for.

It's important to openly recognize and accept that there are opportunities for improvement as you move forward. Practice this with a level of caution. It doesn't do anyone any good for you to beat yourself down about things you did in the past.

Be honest with yourself about any stumbling blocks you have:

- Do I need to improve my note-taking abilities?
- Am I as organized as I should be?
- Am I asking for help when I need it?

The road to self-advocacy is continuous and requires years of continuous learning, tenacity, improvement, and ultimately trial and error.

Don't expect to be perfect. The truth is that just by making an effort to play an active role in your healthcare experience, you are ahead of the game.

IN THIS CHAPTER

» Clearly defining team roles and care objectives

» Encouraging transparent interactions

» Celebrating wins as a team

» Cultivating collaborative decision-making

Chapter 10
Assembling Your Healthcare Allies

Building and cultivating relationships with a reliable support team is essential to navigating your healthcare journey successfully. Whether you're dealing with chronic conditions or just wanting to get the most out of your regular checkups, understanding how to choose, work with, and leverage healthcare professionals is important.

In this chapter I share strategies and tips on how to build a game-winning healthcare roster and how to identify the right doctors and support personnel you need to be on your side to help effectively manage your needs. You explore ways to keep your support system strong and get the most out of your experience with the healthcare system.

Determining Who Should Be on Your Team

Welcome to the healthcare jungle — one of the most daunting and confusing industries to navigate! In all seriousness, the healthcare industry represents not only a vital service and commitment to the management, prevention, and ratification of illness, it's also a multi-billion dollar business. It includes a soup of diverse roles and job functions that are each tailored to ensure equitable, cost effective, and innovative healthcare. This ranges from general practitioners to specialized surgeons, from nurses to hospital administrators, and everything in between.

Amidst its complexity, one of the keys to having a successful healthcare experience is to find the right team to present the facts you need to make decisions about your health, empower you to do so, cheer you on, and steer you in the right direction. Get ready to simplify this thing called healthcare!

Primary care providers: The cornerstone of your well-being

A primary care provider (or physician), also often referred to as the PCP, family doctor, or general practitioner, should be your main point of contact for all of your healthcare needs. This clinical provider should serve as the "clinical quarterback" of your healthcare. This clinician provides preventative care, gives annual physicals, manages chronic health conditions, refers you to specialists when necessary, and more.

Primary care providers are different than specialists, as they have broad knowledge of different conditions and treatments and the training and understanding to know when a specialist needs to be involved in your care. Primary care providers coordinate your overall care, keeping tabs on your overall state of being.

These clinicians can also save patients money when they regularly see them. Seeing a primary care provider on a regular basis can increase your chances of identifying a complex or chronic condition. They can pull in the appropriate team members to address the issue and often nip things in the bud. For example, they are often the first on the care team to notice changes in your baseline condition and diagnose high blood pressure and help patients address this through medication or dietary changes.

WHAT'S IN A NAME?

Wondering why many healthcare professionals use the term "provider" when referring to members of your care team? It's because many patients receive care, such as primary care, from nurse practitioners (NP, FNP, ANP, etc.) and physician's assistants (PA, PA-C, and APA-C), instead of a doctor (MDs or DOs), on a regular basis.

These providers have completed specialized training, graduate education (often to the master and doctoral levels), and certifications to become qualified to see patients, diagnose issues, treat problems, prescribe medication, and more, under the supervision of a physician.

In some places, providers like nurse practitioners can practice independently of doctors. You can read more about nurse practitioners and PAs later in this chapter.

When you regularly see your PCP, you are more likely to:

- **Address a health concern early.** By catching issues early, you can reduce your predisposition to some of the life-threatening complications.
- **Save money on your healthcare spend.** The out-of-pocket cost, or co-pay, you pay to see your PCP is likely much smaller than waiting and then having to see a specialist because your problem has grown in scale and complexity.
- **Improve your quality of life.** When you attend your annual wellness exams and take your PCP's advice, you are more likely to be healthy and fit.

Harnessing expertise: specialists, surgeons, and more

While primary care providers help clinical well-being, specialists and surgeons complete specialized training and have expertise in a very particular area of healthcare, like cardiology, immunology, oncology, or pulmonology. If you are experiencing illnesses that affect a specific part of your body, your PCP may refer you to a specialist to help evaluate the issue and provide you expert care. Some specialists also perform surgery — like cardiac surgeons, neurosurgeons, and orthopedic surgeons.

REMEMBER

Many specialists endure long years of training to become experts in their field. Along the way, providers may have insights or additional information about other conditions outside of their specialty that can be generally helpful. However, maximize your providers expertise in their field by working closely with them on conditions related to their specialty. See Figure 10-1.

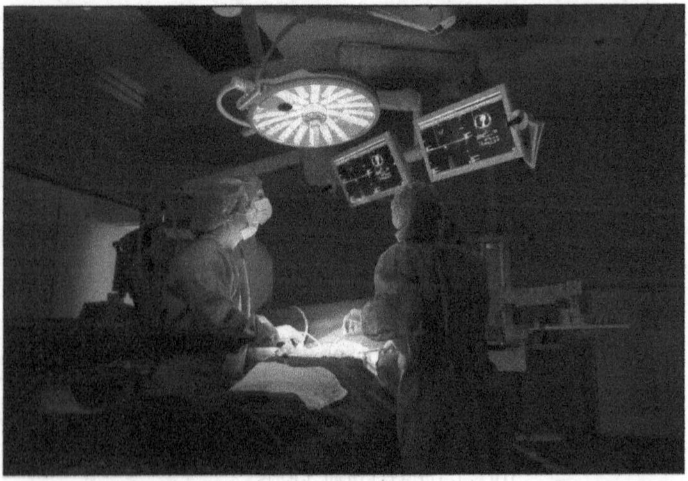

Hispanolistic/Getty Images

FIGURE 10-1: Specialists and surgeons can be referred to you by your primary care physician.

Most providers are very comfortable letting you know when you should see another specialist. However, if for some reason you are not referred to the appropriate specialty, you can ask for a referral.

TIP

For best results, direct your questions about a particular condition to the correct provider. It may be in your best interest to ask your orthopedic surgeon about your knee pain after a knee replacement as opposed to asking your cardiologist. If you don't know who to ask, you can mention it to the provider you're seeing at that moment.

The only "dumb question" is the one you don't ask!

Working with pharmacists

Pharmacists are qualified to maximize medication management and advice. Having a good relationship with your pharmacist can make a significant difference in managing your medication.

Beyond their extensive knowledge of pharmacology, pharmacists are invaluable resources when it comes to answering your questions about proper dosage, potential interactions with other medications, side effects, and so much more.

While they may not be directly involved in your medical care on a regular basis, they have a wealth of information and experience that can help you navigate medication management. They can also champion patient safety by helping identify harmful medication interactions and errors in dosing.

TIP

Pharmacists are often aware of programs, discounts, and other resources to make your medication affordable. Don't be afraid to ask your pharmacist about ways to save money on prescriptions.

In some cases, your pharmacist may be able to start the conversation with your care team about prescribing a generic medication to keep expenses low. They also can help you understand the drug plan component of your insurance coverage and can be pivotal partners in helping you identify the most cost-effective way to afford your medication. They can also connect you with the appropriate contacts, like your formulary at your insurance company, to help you further.

Nurses, nurse practitioners, nurse's aides, and the provision of essential care

Often referred to as the "backbone of the healthcare system," nurses are the everyday heroes who play an extremely essential role on your healthcare team. They often bridge the gap and improve relationships between patients and doctors.

Outside of their clinical duties, nurses often act as patient advocates. They provide emotional, educational, and clinical support to the patients they serve. In many cases — especially in the hospital, in post-op from a surgical procedure, or in the emergency department — patients spend more time interacting with their nurse than they do with their clinician.

Physical and occupational therapists

Physical and occupational therapists (PTs and OTs, respectively) are clinical professionals who have been trained to help patients regain and improve their mobility. They are your partners on the road to rehabilitation and pain management.

- **Physical therapists** focus on the improvement of physical function and the prevention of further disability (such as learning to walk with better mobility after a hip replacement). You might find yourself working with a physical therapist when you're in-patient admitted to the hospital.
- **Occupational therapists** focus on helping patients more effortlessly complete everyday living activities (such as fine motor skills needed to button a coat or raise a fork).

Social workers

Social workers serve as allies in navigating support services and other resources. They are specially trained to help navigate challenges that affect patients' lives outside of clinical care, such as like social welfare issues (food or housing insecurity).

The journey to wellness is a holistic process and not every patient has the same advantages or opportunities to achieve it. Some patient populations, such as those who are low-income, have children and families, or have significant mental or physician disability challenges, struggle navigating major changes in their healthcare journey.

Social workers are knowledgeable about community resources and hospital programs that can help qualified individuals with:

- Pay for a new medication
- Transition from hospitalization to home
- Care coordination in the hospital
- Obtain reliable transportation to their appointments
- Get social and mental health support

Social workers focus on a patient as a whole person, and not just on their health issue. They can be great advocates. Working with social workers can empower you to make good decisions about your healthcare.

REMEMBER

While social workers can offer integral support to patients navigating the healthcare system, they perform a different type of work than private or independent patient advocates. Generally, social workers are employees of the hospital or the health system. They can help patients navigate the complexity of their care within the health system by connecting them with the appropriate resources, gathering additional information about financial assistance, and more.

REMEMBER

Private or independent patient advocates provide patient advocacy services independent of a healthcare system and are often contracted or hired directly by the patient and their family to provide personalized assistance, regardless of where the patient is receiving care.

Consider this example:

Jeff is caring for his aging father, Henry, who is experiencing cognitive changes and was admitted to the hospital after falling in his kitchen and breaking his shoulder. While admitted to the hospital, Jeff worked closely with Henry's social worker, Michelle, to help coordinate his care, ask questions about their case, become aware of resources available to them, and get his father the care he needs.

Michelle has been extremely helpful to Jeff and Henry and made the hospital experience much easier to navigate. After a few days in the hospital, Henry is being discharged home. During the last meeting with the hospitalist before he was sent home, the doctor recommended that Jeff look into long-term care options, like assisted living, for his father.

Having never had the conversation with his father and unsure where to start, Jeff does some research about the considerations that go into the transition of living arrangements, the differences between assisted living, independent living, and long-term care, and how to afford it.

Right before Henry's discharge, Jeff speaks with Michelle about the conversation he had with his father's doctor and begins to ask questions about how to navigate these unchartered waters with his father after discharge. Although Michelle has been helpful and wants to continue helping, unfortunately, Henry is being discharged from the health system and she cannot support their case as intimately as she would like to like she was when he was admitted into the hospital, because they are going home.

She's able to provide Jeff and Henry with some resources about where to start. However, there's still so much for Jeff and Henry to learn and navigate.

Social workers and private advocates are both committed to empowering patients and providing them information to support their decisions. However, in this scenario, Jeff and Henry would best benefit from the guidance of a private or independent professional patient advocate to help them navigate Henry's healthcare journey after discharge.

If Jeff and Henry decide to hire a private advocate, that person could go with Henry wherever he goes and would not be constrained to the jurisdiction of a health system because they are employed independently by Jeff and Henry and not by a healthcare institution.

Mental health professionals

Mental health professionals are experts at addressing psychological and emotional needs. Having mental professional, like a therapist, counselor, psychologist, or psychiatrist, on your team is just as crucial as having a primary care provider, specialized surgeon, or nurse.

The road to wellness, or even just the journey to an improved quality of life, can be extremely taxing. Mental health providers are dedicated to improving your emotional well-being and offer resources to help build your emotional resiliency through life's challenging moments.

Therapists and counselors provide a safe space to discuss your feelings and focus on helping you manage your stress, anxiety, and depression. Psychiatrists are specialized physicians who are trained to diagnose and treat mental health disorders and prescribe medications when needed. Psychologists may use in-depth assessments and techniques to help you gain a better understanding of yourself and a familiarity with your cognitive patterns and behaviors.

You may think that you have all the social support you need to manage your feelings about your healthcare and your healthcare journey in your family and friends. Social support from people you love and care about is great, but working closely with specialized providers who have completed extensive training and certification and have a commitment to mental health can especially help you stay mentally healthy and resilient to endure your healthcare journey.

Caregivers, friends, and family

Your caregivers, friends, and family can be the cheer squad you need. They can serve as a supportive network and keep you encouraged, happy, and accountable to your healthcare journey. Every patient's person social network looks different — some patients may have a multitude of friends and family to support them along their journey, while others have a much smaller close knit community. However, the impact can be great regardless of the size. Caregivers can support daily activities like personal care, medications, and cleaning. Friends and family can share in laughter, be great sounding boards for concerns, and a great diversion on a hard day.

Caregivers, friends, and families don't just get an honorable mention on your healthcare team roster; they have their own unique and impactful place. Family and friends are often ready to be a support to you in the capacity that you need them. Whether they cook dinner for you every week, run a couple errands, or just show up to your doctor's appointments and hold your hand (see Figure 10-2), their contribution is significant, enriching, and needed.

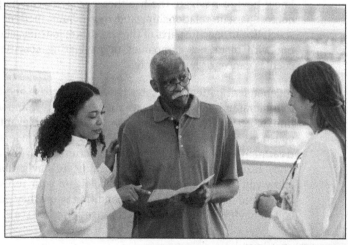

SDI Productions/Getty Images

FIGURE 10-2: Caregivers and family members can be a critical part of your healthcare team if you let them.

TIP

If you don't have the social support of friends and family, consider finding community in other patients who share the same or similar condition. You can find groups from your doctor's office or striking up a conversation in the waiting room with another patient you see all the time or join an online community online for patients who share the same condition. You never know — you might develop a new friend, find a carpool buddy, gain an accountability partner, or just make a friendly acquaintance to wave at periodically.

Don't set expectations for what the interaction should look like or what you want out of that relationship. Social support in community is like a bouquet of flowers — all flowers may not be the same, but together they make something beautiful.

Independent patient advocates

One of the most powerful allies you can have in managing your healthcare is an independent or private patient advocate. These professionals come from a variety of backgrounds. Some are former nurses, physicians, social workers, and certified professional patient advocates (like board-certified patient advocates (BCPAs)). They can be your dedicated point person who ensures that your voice is heard and your needs are met throughout the course of your medical journey.

Patient advocates are specialists in patient rights, and they also know how to navigate the healthcare system, can help with the doctor-patient relationship, and more. Some patient advocates specialize in specific parts of the healthcare journey, such as dealing with insurance companies or navigating specific journeys, such as cancer or hospice care.

Independent patient advocates have the expertise and bandwidth to understand your current situation, your goals, and your timeline for action. They provide you with all of the relevant resources you need to make complex medical decisions, understand your treatment options, or communicate better with your care team. They take the guesswork out of healthcare navigation and can allow you the opportunity to focus solely on your recovery, well-being, and management of your condition while they partner with you to navigate the often-time confusing healthcare system.

TIP

Hiring an independent patient advocate can be one of the best decisions you make. However, they can be a financial investment. Use reputable resources and directories to look for independent or private patient advocates in your area (or ones that travel or work remotely) and identify a few of them that provide the type of support you're looking for!

Keeping Your Support System Strong

Having a support system that is responsive, interactive, complete, and ready to take on the world is like having a brand-new car. The car runs smoothly, it's efficient, and has minimal to no mechanical issues. It feels really good to drive and you know that no matter how far you need to go, your new car can get you there.

How do you ensure that the new "car" continues performing well? If you never change the oil, rotate at the tires, refill the tank, or have it tuned up, the performance of the car will suffer, and eventually the whole unit will break down. Then, you end up spending time and money addressing the repairs to get the car running again.

Your support system is no different. In this section, you learn ways to maintain and strengthen your support system so that continuously uplifts, empowers, and guides you.

Expressing gratitude and appreciation

Gratitude can be a game changer when it comes to your healthcare journey. Having an attitude of gratitude doesn't just strengthen your relationships, it also creates a positive environment for all. The best part is that expressing your gratitude is extremely simple and free!

Here are some ways to thank those who have supported you:

» **Just say thank you.** I know this sounds simple, but saying these two words can have a huge impact. Whether you say thank you to your nurse for sending you a extra package of graham crackers in the emergency department, send a thank you text message to your friend who took you to an early morning MRI, or toss a smile and a thankful hand gesture, small expressions of thanks show that you appreciate someone's efforts. Gratitude can lift the spirit of those who have a vested interest in helping you.

- **Extend a small gesture of appreciation.** Pay attention to the things that your support team likes. You don't have to buy anyone's affection or support with gifts, but writing a thank you note, baking a batch of cookies, or another small gesture can make that person feel special.
- **Acknowledge their efforts.** Give credit where it's due. Even for those who are experienced navigating the healthcare system, it can be tough and sometimes clinicians spend hours trying to identify diagnoses or diseases, create a suitable treatment plan, navigate insurance considerations, and so much more. Go the extra mile and let your healthcare team know that you appreciate their hard work, their commitment, and going the extra mile for you. Acknowledging their efforts allows them to be seen and recognized.

Building trust

Trust is the cornerstone of any healthy relationship. While navigating the world of healthcare, it's important to be able to trust the key members of your team. Trust doesn't magically happen — it has to be built and cultivated, and it requires a commitment to openness and honesty. To build a strong foundation of trust within your support team, you need to make sure that you are exemplifying honesty as well.

To build trust, you have to be transparent and lay all your cards out on the table. There are very few things more personal to a person than their healthcare, their quality of life, and their pursuit of longevity. Because these conversations are very personal, it's understandable to feel guarded. Make a conscious effort to share all relevant information about your health and your condition with your healthcare team.

This information can include:

- Concerns you have about your health
- Social habits that affect your illness or care

» Health habits that affect your illness or care
» Presentation of symptoms

In order for everyone to be on the same page, they need to know all the facts. There shouldn't be any shame in your game. Even though some conditions may feel awkward or embarrassing, professionals in the healthcare system see them, navigate them, and work through them every day. Better to have too much information than not enough.

Communicating clearly

In addition to being transparent and honest, there should be an expectation to communicate clearly. It's your responsibility to ask clarifying questions if you don't understand something. It's also your responsibility to be direct in your communication and to answer any questions your care team has about the information you share with them. This street goes both ways, so make a commitment to direct communication.

REMEMBER

You — and your support team — are human, and mistakes happen. Foster a culture that acknowledges mistakes and works together to find solutions. Mistakes are scary; however, what's scarier is mistrust. Acknowledge the humanity of your team by making a conscious effort to provide feedback about why something didn't work, how it could be done better, and what to do as a team if it happens again.

Understanding and respecting roles, responsibilities, and boundaries

Everybody on your support team is essential to the collective mission of pursuing your wellness. By the same token, everyone's contribution and role is different.

Consider the following tips for respecting everyone's roles and maximizing their impact:

» **Make it your business to know your team.** Just like an orchestra has a conductor and musicians who play different instruments and have specific roles, your healthcare team is made up of a multitude of professionals with their own expertise and responsibilities. From doctors who diagnose conditions to pharmacists who help you manage your medication, every person plays a part in making music.

TIP

Familiarize yourself with the roles and responsibilities of each person on your team. This helps manage your expectations. If you don't know the role or even title of a professional you are working with, ask! New members of your clinical team should identify themselves when they walk into your exam room or reach out to you. If they do not (or if you didn't hear or understand them), ask them how their role interacts with your care.

- **Be respectful of each professional's boundaries.** Each professional has boundaries around the type and amount of care that they can provide, given their training and their role on your care team. As you learn the responsibilities of the professionals you are working with, respect their limits. Don't ask them, or expect them, to perform functions outside of their job. For example, it's not within the scope of practice of a registered nurse (RN) to diagnose patients. That's something your doctor, nurse practitioner, or physician assistant could do.

  Respecting their roles allows everyone to work within their strengths, training, and expertise and ensures that they're able to support you.

- **Coordinate and collaborate as a unit.** Look at every interaction with a healthcare professional as a chance to coordinate and collaborate. If your healthcare journey is a ship, you should be the captain. It's your responsibility to ask questions if you're unsure about why someone does what they do, who else needs to be part of the conversation, and what you can expect. Clinical providers and healthcare professionals are used to working in team dynamics — on the front lines to serve the patient, as well as behind the scenes administratively and operationally — so asking a member of your care team who else needs to get pulled in is okay. Ensuring that everyone's efforts are harmonized, appropriate, and dynamic positions you for the best outcome.

Familiarizing yourself with the rules of each health professional on your team, working together to respect their boundaries, and coordinating, communicating, and collaborating as a unit can build a dynamic and resilient support system that will allow you to navigate whatever is ahead.

Addressing Conflicts Professionally

Even the most efficient, effective, and collaborative teams experience turbulence and conflicts. Conflicts may be caused by miscommunication, one party not feeling heard or respected, lack of resources, and a plethora of other issues. Conflict is normal and will happen. Navigating conflict effectively means managing your approach, expectations, and accountability. With a bit of diplomacy and understanding, you can handle stressful scenarios like a pro.

The following sections describe some tips for addressing conflicts professionally.

Get to the bottom of the problem

To properly address the conflict, you need to start by identifying what spurred it. Were expectations mismanaged? Was a mistake made on the team and not owned?

Start by taking inventory of what you know and the perspective of those affected. Take a page from *Dragnet*'s Sergeant Joe Friday, and tell yourself "all [you] want are the facts!".

TIP

When finding facts about the root cause of a conflict, approach the situation with curiosity, and not with judgment or prejudice, to get a sense for what's going on. You're human and it makes sense to have your own preconceived opinion of what's going on. However, if you don't keep your perspective in check, you can bias your investigation and overlook or omit factors that impacted the situation and caused the conflict.

Prioritize clear and open communication

Consider the adage: "You have two ears and one mouth, so you should listen twice as much as you speak." Create an environment where all parties feel comfortable and safe communicating their side of the story or perspective. It's important to approach each conversation with empathy and be genuinely willing to listen. No one is expecting you not to feel emotions like anger, disappointment, and frustration. However, it's important to share your perspective in a calm, respectful manner.

To solve these issues, try these approaches:

- Gather all the facts.
- Find common ground between you and everybody involved.
- Create a safe and respectful environment for everyone to openly communicate their perspectives.
- Shift your attention to identifying common interests and goals.
- Look for a middle ground and realign the group to what's important.

Suddenly, the conversation is focused on solutions instead of differences. This sets the stage for the "What do we do next?" or "How do we avoid this in the future?" conversations and allows everyone to set clear expectations of future engagements.

After the conflict is resolved, touch base with members of your team to:

- Determine how the resolution went
- See if other challenges have popped up
- Ensure that everyone feels valued and heard

REMEMBER

It the patient's responsibility to take the initiative and be an active participant in their care — even when the waters get choppy. In order to receive the patient-centered, individualized care, support, and resources you seek, everything — including conflict resolution — has to be personalized. Don't wait for a doctor, social worker, or other member of your team to take the initiative and start solving problems.

WARNING

If the conflict you are faced with involves harm, unprofessionalism that can't be managed between you and your healthcare professionals, negligence, or some other serious issue, you don't have to lead the charge alone. Resources like the hospital ombudsman, patient advocate, or other members of health system leadership are available and can hold the appropriate parties accountable. It helps to know about these resources and who to talk to if you need them.

If necessary, ask someone you trust to sit in as a neutral third party during conflict resolution. This way, you have the perspective of someone not intimately involved or affected by the conflict. This person could be a close friend or another healthcare professional you trust, just to name a couple.

Set clear, achievable expectations

Set expectations with your support system to ensure that everyone is on the same page and can move forward as a unit. When you set clear expectations, everyone understands what they are responsible for, how their efforts contribute to your overall care and well-being, how to mitigate similar concerns in the future, and how you expect support.

Look for the lesson

Study how the conflict arose and how it was mitigated. Identify ways to make your support system more dynamic. Conflict can serve as an opportunity to learn. Frame your thinking so that every bump in the road presents you with an opportunity to grow and become more resilient.

As you and your team work together along your healthcare journey, you won't feel like you're putting out fires as much as addressing conflicts head-on with a strategic, streamlined approach. You'll be fostering resilience among your team members.

REMEMBER

Conflict is normal. Your involvement in addressing it is crucial to the quality of the care you receive. Your well-being is worth it.

Celebrating Small Successes Together

It's important to take a pause and appreciate your victories along the way:

- That time when you figured out how to log in to your online health management app? That is a win.
- Using the reminder app on your phone to finally schedule your medication? That's a win.

Each step you take along your journey is a building block toward the achievement of a larger goal. Sometimes, we focus so intensely on achieving the big goals. There's nothing wrong with striving to achieve large goals; however, don't underestimate the impact of the smaller foundational goals that those larger ones are built on.

Celebrating the small wins with your support system and your clinical care team not only strengthens the connection between you and the members of your team, but it also contributes to the positive, collaborative atmosphere and the realization that you are making progress.

Consider the following tips to celebrate every win, no matter how modest they may seem, and give them the recognition they deserve.

Acknowledge every milestone

Every step you take along your journey of completing a marathon is just as important as crossing the finish line. In many parts of life, not just in navigating the healthcare system, people make a laundry list of goals or events they want to achieve and focus so intensely on them that they have trouble appreciating the completion of goals and milestones that are not as "major."

- Lowering your blood pressure slightly is just as meaningful as lowering it to the point where you don't need to take medication.
- Having a day with less pain than normal is just as important as going a day without feeling any pain at all.

Every win is worth celebrating. When you adopt that mindset and share your wins with other members of your support system, not only are you encouraged with reminders about your progress and how resilient you are, but your support system is also encouraged.

Intentionally celebrate your successes

Celebrate by doing something that you enjoy, by taking a break from your normal day, or by doing something you would typically save for a special occasion. Get your nails done or watch tonight's game with your friend at a restaurant.

Learn to congratulate yourself on making progress or sticking to a goal by practicing the celebratory rituals you normally save for big events.

TIP

Bonus points if you celebrate these wins with people in your support system. Maybe you take a family member who has been serving as your accountability partner out for dinner or you drop your clinical care team a note about your progress.

Have a "wins" report-out

When a team finishes an initiative or a project, they "report out" relevant information to other members of their team, their leadership, and or other relevant stakeholder of their organization. The report out usually includes an overview of the process, their successes, their opportunities for improvement, and, and their vision going forward.

At your next doctor's appointment — when you are giving a "report out" to your team about how you've been managing your condition, what's been working, what's not working, areas for improvement, and other relevant information — add a section to talk about your wins and make an effort to always report at least one win to your team.

This doesn't have to be an elaborate report and can take a couple seconds to a minute, depending on how much you want to share. Believe it or not, one of the biggest reasons that healthcare professionals go into and stay in the healthcare field is because they genuinely want to help people get better. Hearing about what's working for you and how you celebrated it lifts everyone's spirits. You will feel like you accomplished something, and your care team will appreciate hearing about it.

Feature a mini appreciation award moment

Try this at your next clinical appointment. After the report out of your wins, recognize your clinical team in a heartfelt way by taking note of the small gestures or problems they solved that made your life easier.

You could create different "award categories" and give an honorable mention or a shout-out to each member of your team. If you are a crafty person, you could write a personalized note or create a paper award with different themes for each category and then present them to members of your support team.

Maybe the front desk scheduler at your doctor's office was able to get you a last-minute appointment, so at the appointment, you present them with the "Scheduling Savant" award.

Let's say your pharmacist identified a possible drug interaction between the new medication you're starting and a medication you've been taking for a long time. It sounds like they would be a landslide winner for the "Drug Interaction Insight Champion" award!

Recognizing these small, but mighty, actions can really add up. Bonus tip — don't forget to recognize yourself!

If anyone deserves to wear the "World's Most Resilient Patient" pin, it's you!

Navigating Tomorrow's Health as a Team

Your health journey is forever changing — new diagnoses, symptoms, medications, administrative burdens, information, and more. The approach you take to support your care needs to be dynamic and responsive in order to navigate any new challenges that arise. This section discusses some tips for building a plan that can change as you do.

Stay informed

Stay informed about new diagnoses you've received, new treatments available on the market, important insurance information, and any other areas that affect your care.

Make a commitment to continued education and learning about factors that will ultimately affect your care. This sets a precedent with your care team that you are invested and involved in your care, and it encourages your providers and care team to be that way as well.

This doesn't mean you have to make all these decisions alone. When you know about the latest treatments or medications, for example, you are better poised to ask your care team about these breakthroughs and discuss whether they might be good for you.

Review and revise your health goals regularly

To make sure your goals are still relevant, realistic, and achievable, you need to review them on a regular basis. Work with each member of your support system to revise your health goals so that are directly aligned with the support and care you need. See Figure 10-3.

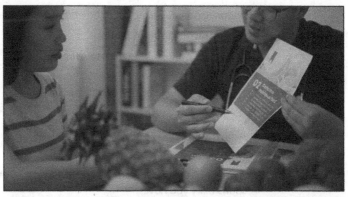

Graphicscoco/Getty Images

FIGURE 10-3: Be sure to revise your health goals as your condition changes.

TIP

Sometimes you will experience changes in different aspects of your healthcare journey all at one time. To keep organized, take notes in a dedicated space about changes in your health or your journey. As you notice things or get new information, make note of this and set a reminder to discuss these changes with the appropriate members of your care team. Also note the plan of action moving forward.

As always, make sure your team and providers understand your concerns and that you are all on the same page.

Prioritize your self-care

Be intentional with the habits and practices you adopt. Navigating the healthcare system, especially with limited to no support, is extremely exhausting. You not only have to actively manage your care, but you also have to keep all members of your team accountable, and stay on the lookout for new and evolving information about your condition.

REMEMBER

Make time for important parts of your life outside of your healthcare journey, like spending time with family and friends, working, resting and relaxing, and so much more. Take time now and then to inventory how you feel, and give yourself an opportunity to rest, recharge, manage stress, exercise, and eat healthy. If you don't, you will burn out, and no one wants that.

Prioritizing self-care can means different things to different people:

- Scheduling one day a month to do nothing
- Spending time walking in nature
- Silencing your phone after a certain time at night so you can get enough sleep
- Practicing mindfulness for a couple minutes
- Petting your dog or cat
- Brushing your teeth before you go to bed
- Taking a long, hot shower or bath
- Booking a 14-day vacation to Fiji and unplugging from every responsibility you have

Whatever that means for you, identify ways to do it and plan to be accountable.

TIP

You can share your plan to prioritize your care with your support system and use others as accountability partners. Maybe that means asking your significant other to remind you to where the compression socks your clinician asked you to wear before you go to work in the morning, or asking your neighbor to take a walk with you around the block every Tuesday so you can be more active.

Prioritize prevention

You can do this by working with your care team to identify risks to current treatment plans and conditions as well as future ones.

Consider this scenario:

Kayla, a very busy mom of three, finds out that she has elevated cholesterol levels at her annual wellness visit. She has a family history of cardiovascular disease, so she realizes that it would be helpful to identify risk factors that could contribute to the onset of a cardiovascular disease in the future. Working with her team, she identifies some lifestyle changes she can make to improve her heart health.

She gets a decent amount of exercise because her family keeps her busy, but she realizes she needs to be more intentional about adhering to a heart-healthy diet. She focuses on making healthier meals that she can meal prep at home and package for on-the-go travel instead.

Consider these tips for creating a prevention plan:

- **Identify all your risks.** To be an informed and empowered consumer of the healthcare system, practice asking what will happen if you do or do not take a recommended action.

  Ask your providers to review all risk factors relevant to you, including ones that you may be genetically predisposed to. Having all the cards on the table allows you to understand the various scenarios.

- **Identify resources to support your prevention plan.** Creating a robust prevention plan is a powerful step in the right direction, but to make it actionable, you need to identify any resources at your disposal that can help make the implementation and sustainability of a prevention plan manageable and effective. Efforts to prevent additional illness and risks are only helpful if you use them. Take inventory of the resources you have to support your plan.

- **Ask your healthcare providers for referrals.** That way, you can see specialists who can provide you additional insights about your condition.

  Sometimes, when a patient and their care team identifies a health condition that could present a problem in the future, they put an initial plan in place to help lower the risk of developing it, like pre-diabetes. If the preventative plan doesn't work as well as anticipated, and the patient begins to develop the condition, they may have the opportunity to work with a specialist to help them manage specific health risks.

» **Become familiar with your community health resources.** Community centers may offer programs like health screenings, food assistance programs, free or low cost fitness classes, and more, which support parts of your health plan. Being aware of community health resources can keep your costs down.

» **Leverage health apps and technology to remind you of important parts of your prevention plan and track progress.** These apps track how many calories you intake, how many calories you burn, the rise and fall of your insulin levels, health appointments, and more. Spend a little bit of time cross-referencing which parts of your prevention plan can be supported by technology and look into different apps that could assist you. Check the reviews and play around with their platforms to see how user friendly they are. You can also use free trials of premium packages.

» **Connect with others at support groups who share your mission or prevention plan.** Being a part of a community of people who share similar health goals and conditions may allow you to learn about different ways to achieve the same goal. You get perspectives and recommendations on what works and what doesn't. This can also build a sense of camaraderie. Local support groups may be available at your hospital system, at nearby universities, or even online. See Figure 10-4.

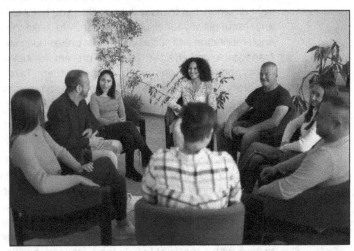

Vladimir Vladimirov/E+/Getty Images

FIGURE 10-4: A support group can give patients the opportunity to connect with others on a similar health journey.

TIP

One size does not fit all, so approach support groups with an open mind. Some people like to be a part of a community where everyone shares a common interest or illnesses, while others would rather work with their care team and make progress as an individual.

Remember, advice and recommendations that you receive from a support group, although helpful and well-intentioned, may not be relevant to your specific healthcare journey, so do your own research, and run the recommendations by your provider.

Establish communication protocols

Make sure everyone on your care team knows the most effective method for communicating within the team and with you.

Communication should be open, clear, concise, and purposeful. This is important when you are planning the success of your future health. Take time to evaluate the most effective way to communicate long-term goals with each member of your care team.

Ask yourself, "What do I want my health to look like in six months? Twelve months? Two years?" You don't have to have all of the answers, or even a general idea right now, but it may benefit you to put a vague picture together of where you would like to be at certain points in time, given the information you've collected with your team.

TIP

Have a check-in conversation every few months and ask your provider and care team their opinions about how feasible your goals are. Make an intentional effort to have a review session of what's worked, what's not worked, what's going on, and what needs to happen to meet certain objectives in the next three to six months, or over several years.

Use this time to listen to the perspectives of those who have been navigating your healthcare journey alongside you and identify goals, plans, and objectives you want to meet as well as the communication method you will use to troubleshoot problems and report progress. For some issues, it may be best to meet face to face at a clinical appointment, but with others a phone call will do.

Ask your team what their preferred method of communication is to talk about future health planning. Each member of your team performs a different function and has varying degrees of bandwidth.

However frequently you meet to discuss, make sure that the interaction invites a meaningful conversations with an emphasis on actionable objectives and problem solving. These plans are dynamic, meaning that they need to be able to respond to the changing environment of your healthcare appropriately.

TIP

When scheduling semiannual health planning meetings, call the office and schedule a 45-minute appointment instead of a 20-minute appointment that you usually have, which allows ample time for conversation. If this is not an option, ask for alternatives.

Coordinating Your Specialized Healthcare Teams

Every specialized team is like a piece of a puzzle. They have their own identity and illuminate part of the picture, but in collaboration and when interlocking with other pieces, the whole picture is revealed.

You can have multiple healthcare specialists on your team that focus on a specific aspect of your health. Your cardiologist works to improve your heart, your psychologist or therapist partners with you to achieve mental well-being, and your gastroenterologist may focus on your gut health. These specialists and their specialist teams have completed rigorous educational requirements and dedicated years of practice to becoming experts in their specialty.

Knowing the roles and objectives of each team member helps you better coordinate their efforts. It's your responsibility to have a bird's-eye view of how each team works, what their mission is, their goals, and how they can collaborate in conversations about your total health and well-being. See Figure 10-5.

Think of your team as a large organization and you are the chief executive officer (CEO). Each specialist is the head of their own department and they focus on a specific process, operation, or service.

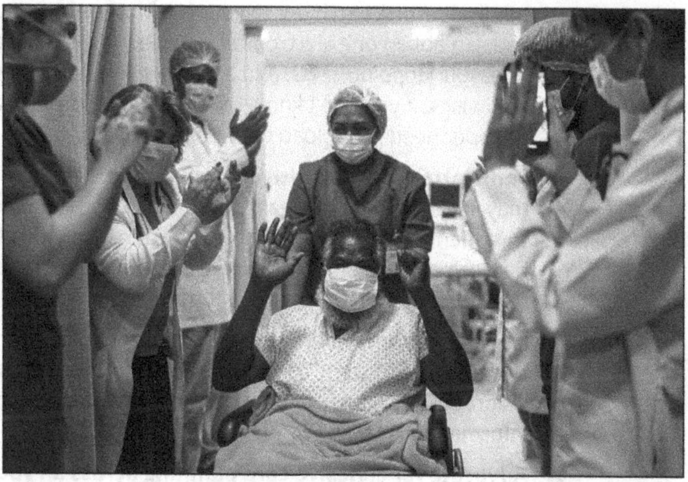

FG Trade/Getty Images

FIGURE 10-5: A great healthcare team feels your wins as strongly as you do.

As the CEO of your healthcare, it's your responsibility to make sure that every part of the "business" is collectively working together to achieve your North Star objectives.

In the healthcare environment, those objectives could be things like finding the right diagnosis, finding affordable medication, getting you the best care possible, and more.

Here are some tips for helping your care team collaborate and solve overall issues:

- **Take inventory of your team.** Make a list of each specialty and service you interact with across all parts of your care, the main point of contact, the support staff, and what the specialty or service is supposed to help you do. Write down any goals you've made with that particular team, the timeline in which you have agreed to complete things, and an overview of the guidance they provided.
- **Make sure communication from all your providers is recorded in your medical records.** It's impossible to expect everybody to be on the same page if information from one team is not properly or accurately included in your medical records. Providers usually have a time frame as to when they need to upload visit notes to the electronic medical record and for them to be viewable. If you don't have access to your

medical record, reach out to your health system and ask how you can obtain one electronically. Review your medication lists, your appointments, and any other relevant notes from your visits. If you don't know the time frame in which a provider needs to upload their notes, just ask.

- **Familiarize yourself with common medical terms.** You may see certain terms again and again in visit notes and on treatment plans across multiple providers. You don't have to be a pro at understanding everything, but it does help to have understand the common terminology.

  TIP

  If you don't know where to start, turn to Chapter 2, which contains lists of some common medical terms. You can also visit reputable sites, like WebMD or the Mayo Clinic, to find information you can rely on.

- **Advocate for cohesive care planning across all your teams.** Even though providers and clinical teams are used to working with other multi-disciplinary teams to ensure that they are holistically treating a patient, it never hurts to discuss your healthcare goals and make your wants known. Make your providers aware of the other types of specialists you are working with. You can also ask for recommendations on what other teams need to be brought into conversation about your health regarding the specific condition they are treating. For example, when a patient is being treated for cancer and experiences other health problems, it's not uncommon for their oncologist to still be in the loop of their care.

Each team in your support system must work well together. The collective goal is your overall health and wellness. It's your responsibility to play an active role in orchestrating team harmony and collaboration. You're not alone on your healthcare journey; you have allies and specialists to help. Creating a supportive, respectful, collaborative environment allows every member of the team to achieve those specific and holistic health goals, with you at the center.

4

Confronting Healthcare Headwinds

IN THIS PART . . .

Handling misdiagnoses and getting second opinions

Dealing with health insurance coverage gaps and tackling medical debt

Planning for the evolving needs of chronic and long-term conditions

Avoiding infection and mitigating medical harm by prioritizing your personal safety

IN THIS CHAPTER

» Understanding the common causes of misdiagnoses

» Handling the emotional and physical consequences of misdiagnosis

» Minimizing misdiagnoses

» Asking for a second opinion

Chapter 11 Navigating Misdiagnoses and Getting Second Opinions

Misdiagnoses are much more common than you might think and they can lead to improper treatment, unnecessary stress, and even prolonged discomfort, symptoms, or disease.

One of the best tools for mitigating misdiagnoses is the second opinion. Whether you're unsure if your diagnosis is correct or just interested in gathering additional insights about your condition, a second opinion can help identify the best treatment plan and potentially provide you peace of mind.

This chapter demystifies the steps you need to take to gather essential information and take steps in the right direction toward confirming a proper diagnosis and beginning the path to recovery.

Understanding the Impact of Misdiagnoses

Saying that a misdiagnosis can mess things up is an understatement. Misdiagnoses not only affect patients physically by way of a less-than-optimal treatment plan, incorrect treatment plan, or prolonged disease, but they can also have emotional effects.

There are many reasons that patients experience a misdiagnosis. The following sections break down why misdiagnoses happen, the emotional and physical fallout, and how to avoid them. By homing in on the specific points, patients can be better prepared to address the possibility of misdiagnosis, leading to a more informed and potentially better healthcare experience.

Common causes of misdiagnoses

Here are some of the most common reasons behind misdiagnoses.

- **Miscommunication between the patient and clinician.** This can set both parties up for failure. Sometimes, what a patient says and what a doctor hears are entirely different.

  REMEMBER

  You can avoid miscommunication by keeping your responses and storytelling clear and concise, coming to your doctor's appointment prepared with talking points you want to address, reviewing your doctor's clinical note in your medical record, and escalating any discrepancies in your story. If possible, bring a friend or family member to all of your appointments to be a second set of ears.

- **Limited access to accurate patient medical history.** The clinician then doesn't have a complete picture of the patient's medical background. When important details are missing, misdiagnoses are much more likely.

  TIP

  Be sure that your medical records are transferred if you seeing a provider or doctor outside your home healthcare system. Contact the records department weeks before your appointment to ensure your medical records are transferred in time. Contact the releasing hospital or doctor's office to learn the transfer process. You might need to sign an authorization form to get your records from one provider to another and pay applicable fees. Don't wait until the last minute!

It's important to confirm with both offices which records are being sent and which have been received. This ensures transparency. Fill out authorization forms accurately and completely to avoid any potential misinformation that results in delays. Regularly check the status of the transfer. By the time your appointment arrives, your new clinician will have all the necessary and accurate information to review your case and provide the best possible care.

- **Time constraints during patient consultations and examinations.** Clinicians often have a limited time to spend with each patient, and because of this, information that is important for the workup and, ultimately, the diagnosis can be omitted.
- **Variability in clinical expertise and experiences.** Not all clinicians are created equally. Various levels of expertise and experience can result in different clinical decision-making processes and diagnoses.
- **Cognitive biases and diagnostic oversights.** Even the best clinicians make mistakes. Consider the following types of biases that can happen:

Anchoring bias	Hyper-fixating on the first symptom and paying less attention to other symptoms
Overconfidence bias	Being overconfident in the initial treatment or diagnosis and potentially overlooking critical details
Confirmation bias	Paying attention to symptoms that support the initial diagnosis and ignoring evidence that challenges it
Availability heuristic	Recalling (consciously or otherwise) a recent, similar diagnosis from another patient that fits the symptoms and diagnosing a patient with the same condition even if it's not quite accurate

» Examples include:
- A provider misinterpreting your test results
- Not ordering the proper tests
- Leaving out vital information to make the correct diagnosis
- Rushing a thorough physical exam and missing key signs that are crucial for a correct diagnosis

Some of these opportunities are outside the scope of control for a patient; however, being aware of these potential pitfalls and taking appropriate steps to avoid them can improve diagnostic accuracy, ensure that you receive the best patient outcomes, and reduce the possibility of being misdiagnosed.

Emotional and physical consequences

To put things lightly, misdiagnoses can throw a real curveball into your healthcare journey. They can cause unnecessary medical harm or even cost some patients their lives. Dealing with the added stress and confusion of figuring out what's wrong and how to correct it can take a toll on your physical and emotional well-being.

This section breaks down some of the emotional and physical consequences of being misdiagnosed. The final section talks about ways to minimize the risk of being misdiagnosed.

Delayed treatment and illness progression

For some conditions, like cancer, time is of the essence, and providers need to identify the condition correctly, put together an effective treatment plan, and start interventions as soon as possible. If adequate medical treatment is delayed, it's possible the illness or disease could progress, symptoms could worsen, and the patient's quality of life can be jeopardized. Delayed treatment increases the difficulty of managing a condition and results in complex health problems.

Unnecessary treatments, medications, and side effects

If you don't know what something is, you don't accurately know how to treat it. Being diagnosed with the wrong condition can lead to unnecessary treatments being administered, unnecessary or incorrect medications being prescribed, and unwanted side effects from a treatment plan that doesn't fit the situation. These unnecessary treatments and medications can lead to additional health issues, which are compounded with existing conditions.

Increased stress and anxiety

Increased anxiety and stress can have real physiological impacts on a person's physical health, as well as take a toll emotionally. Constantly waiting for a proper diagnosis, dealing with delays, and taking unnecessary medications and treatments not only increases the stress and anxiety patients feel but can impact the well-being of loved ones and care team members, therefore creating a more tense environment and adding to the burden of illness.

Loss of trust

When a patient experiences an incorrect diagnosis, has to endure unnecessary or ineffective treatments and medications, they will understandably lose trust in their healthcare providers and in the healthcare system. They may become wary of their team's clinical expertise, wonder if their providers have their best interests at heart, or become fearful of their safety and well-being, thinking it could happen again.

Without a trusted relationship, specifically a collaborative, patient-centered healthcare relationship, patients may not comply with treatment plans and may discontinue even seeing their clinician.

TIP

If, for whatever reason, you find yourself losing trust in your clinical care team and you do not see improvement when you talk about your concerns, it's okay to discontinue seeing that provider. Just because a health system assigns you a provider doesn't mean you're forced to continue to follow with them.

Contact your hospital system or provider's office for more information about changing providers. Be sure to ask for a providers in your health insurance network and inquire about the financial impact of making this change, if any.

Increased financial burden

Additional unnecessary appointments and treatments associated with misdiagnoses can contribute to significant financial strain.

Healthcare is already as expensive — let alone when the diagnosis is incorrect. Patients may accumulate additional medical bills, out-of-pocket expenses for prescriptions and treatments, and rising healthcare costs for conditions they're currently managing. They might reach the insurance limits on their annual plan sooner than anticipated, draining their savings or health savings account, and much more.

WARNING

In some cases, misdiagnoses can be considered medical negligence and can prompt the filing of a medical malpractice lawsuit. Damages recovered in these cases could include medical expenses and other related financial damages. Navigating these complex situations requires professional help, so seek advice from a reputable medical malpractice attorney to get the best guidance for your case.

Minimizing the Possibility of Being Misdiagnosed

The goal for everyone on the healthcare team should be to prevent misdiagnoses at all costs. While some factors are beyond your control as the patient or caregiver, such as the thoroughness of the clinical providers, there are many practical things you can do. This section discusses some simple and effective strategies.

Ensure that communication is clear

Communicate everything to your provider as fully, clearly, and concisely as possible. Information you may view as trivial could be critical to your doctor's decision-making process. Make your communication purposeful and brief. Honesty is key in any collaborative relationship. Talk to your clinician about the symptoms you're experiencing, what makes them better, what makes them worse, your habits, and your concerns.

Withholding information won't help you, so rip the band-aid off when possible. You won't make your clinician squeamish or gross them out with details — you'd be surprised by what they're used to hearing.

Maintain an up-to-date, comprehensive medical history

It's your responsibility to ensure that your clinical care team has the most current information about your medical history before and during the appointment. If you are seeing a provider for the first time and have established your care at another hospital, make sure in advance that your medical records are sent in their entirety to the proper department.

Information that your clinician needs includes things like these:

- Previous illnesses
- Surgeries and the dates of these surgeries
- Current medical conditions and diagnoses
- Allergies
- Family history of illnesses
- Medications you're taking

This will provide them with a complete picture of where you've been to help you get to where you need to go.

TIP

Take your medical history communication further and prepare an "elevator pitch" of your current and most recent medical issues and concerns. Before your appointment, write down the following information:

- When your symptoms started
- How they feel
- What makes them better or worse
- Interventions you've tried
- How long you've been experiencing the symptoms
- Whether you have a family history (if known) of similar issues

Ideally, you can communicate a very streamlined version of this information in about 30 seconds.

Remember, your clinical team will ask you clarifying questions as the appointment continues; however, coming prepared to answer some of your clinician's key questions helps get the ball rolling.

Ask clarifying questions

If your clinical provider gave you a diagnosis or introduced a treatment plan that leaves you scratching your head, ask your questions! It's your right to gain a better understanding of your diagnosis and the plan to treat it.

Your clinical team's responsibility is to provide you with that information. After all, this is new information for you, and understandably, you have questions, so don't feel weird about it.

Ask about differential diagnoses

A *differential diagnosis* is a possible condition your provider has identified as the cause for your symptoms. It's not uncommon for providers to have a handful. For example, differential diagnoses for abdominal pain could range from indigestion from the tacos you had last night for dinner to a bowel obstruction. Considering a multitude of diagnoses helps providers rule out incorrect ones and identify the correct diagnosis and treatment plan.

When you're diagnosed with a condition, ask your clinician about the differential diagnosis they're considering with the simple question, "Could it be anything else?" You can ask, "What are your differential diagnoses for my symptoms, and how did you conclude that this is [*insert diagnosis*]?"

At this point, your provider can recall their clinical decision-making and explain why they feel your symptoms best align with the current diagnosis. Listen for their responses on how they ruled out other diagnoses and why they are confident their diagnosis is correct.

Ask about the road ahead

Now that you have a diagnosis, it's important to understand the road ahead. Consider asking your clinician these questions:

- What improvements will you see to your condition once you begin the treatment plan?
- How long will it take for you to see improvement?
- Are there any side-effects to this treatment plan?

» What changes should you look out for that would indicate a problem?

» What kinds of symptoms should prompt you to seek emergency medical attention?

This conversation should be a healthy dialogue between you and your provider about what to expect next.

Build a collaborative culture

Building a mutually respectful and collaborative decision-making culture between you and your clinical care team will make it easier for you to speak up when something doesn't seem right. Prioritize active listening during your clinician's appointments. Chapter 5 talks more about communicating with your clinical care team.

Ask for support

Whether it's from a professional patient advocate, a family member, or a friend, support is key.

The journey through the healthcare system is daunting; however, you don't have to do it alone. Ask a friend or family member to provide moral support during your appointments or to help keep all your facts in order. Consider hiring a private patient advocate if you need someone dedicated to your care.

Telling Your Clinician You Want a Second Opinion

Telling your clinician you want a second opinion can feel awkward. You might think your clinician will be mad at you because you think you're questioning their clinical expertise or don't trust them. This should not be the case. The second opinion is for you and your peace of mind, and a collaborative, supportive provider will understand that.

REMEMBER

Studies have shown that 88 percent of patients who seek a second opinion leave with a refined or changed diagnosis!

At the end of the day, you are trying to make the best decision for your health. Consider these tips when broaching this subject with your care team.

Approach the conversation respectfully and calmly

You don't have to justify yourself to anyone. If you want a second opinion, you have every right to get one. However, many patients want to give their care team a heads-up about their plans. If you feel inclined to, you can provide a very brief caveat as to why you would like a second opinion. For example, you might indicate that you would like to know what other treatment options are available to you that may be less aggressive.

Talking to your provider about getting a second opinion can help you learn the hospital policy regarding second opinions and provide insight into getting one covered by your insurance company, if applicable.

During this conversation, acknowledge that you trust your current provider's expertise (if that's true), but you want another perspective to help you make the best decision.

REMEMBER

You don't owe anyone an explanation. Don't feel you must gain anyone's blessing to get a second opinion. It's your right.

Address potential concerns and reactions

Unfortunately, there's no way to tell how your provider will react to the news that you want to seek a second opinion. Some providers will be overwhelmingly understanding, while others may be defensive or slightly offended that you're considering the thought.

It's important to understand that second opinions are common and that getting another set of eyes on an issue can provide alternative perspectives, solutions, identification of risks, and so much more that is important to the healthcare service you're receiving.

WARNING

If your provider responds in an overly negative way your request, you have every right to end that conversation, the appointment, or even the relationship with the provider. It is your right as a patient to be treated fairly and respectfully by all members of staff. Report unprofessional misconduct to the hospital ombudsman, hospital leadership, or even the state medical board. If a provider becomes triggered by the idea of you seeking a second opinion, you might have bigger issues on your hands.

Seeking Second Opinions

Consider this scenario:

Geneva has been working closely with her doctor to get a diagnosis for a set of symptoms she has been experiencing over the last few weeks. After several appointments, her doctor diagnoses her, but something feels a little off. For some reason, she can't put away this gut feeling that the diagnosis is incorrect. She is considering getting a second opinion but doesn't know where to start.

Rule number one is always to trust your intuition. If you feel like something is off, there's probably a reason. It doesn't necessarily mean that your clinician is wrong; maybe they could have done a better job explaining the diagnosis. Either way, you have the right to get a second opinion to ensure you're moving in the right direction. Good clinicians are not offended by patients who want a second opinion. If you're concerned that your provider will be, you might want to consider whether it's in your best interest to continue seeing that clinician.

When searching for a provider to give you a second opinion, find someone that is among the most qualified specialists in their field. At this point, you have an initial diagnosis that most likely is within the scope of practice of a specialist. For example, some cardiologists specialize in congestive heart failure. If you've been recently diagnosed with congestive heart failure, you can get a second diagnosis from one of these specialists.

TIP

Ask for your imaging and lab results to be reviewed by another specialist to catch potential errors. Radiologists and pathologist are human and they can overlook findings that can be impactful to your diagnosis.

The following sections discuss considerations when identifying a qualified specialist to explore a second opinion.

Research and identify qualified specialists

Once you've received your diagnosis, look for clinicians who specialize in that disease. These providers may have completed fellowships specific to treating populations of patients with that particular disease, have research interests about your condition, and more.

Check out your hospital's website for other providers you're interested in speaking to.

Request referrals from your primary care provider

If you receive a diagnosis from a general healthcare practitioner who doesn't specialize in the condition they believe you have, you can ask them questions like these:

- "If you were diagnosed with this condition, who would you recommend I establish specialized care with?"
- "Is there a specific hospital or department you recommend I contact to learn more about my condition and manage it?"

Some hospitals have centers of excellence, which are specialized teams that focus on a particular area of expertise or condition. They may have several specialists who can provide you an excellent second opinion.

TIP

Some hospitals are leaders in treating specific conditions. For example, health systems may have award-winning or nationally ranked cancer treatment centers. If you've been recently diagnosed, it may be worthwhile to look for someone who specializes in the specific type of cancer.

Verify credentials and review potential specialists

"Shopping" for a doctor is real and something you should be doing (if you're not already). When looking for a potential specialist to provide you with a second opinion, you should ensure that the provider is licensed in the state where they practice.

Certain specialists in a specific field opt to become board-certified. If they are, double-check their board certification, any affiliations they have with larger hospitals, especially if they're in private practice, and how many years they've been practicing medicine.

You can reach out to friends and contacts for their opinions. Joining a disease-specific social group on social media can provide insights as well, as many other patients are also looking for the best providers to treat their condition. Everyone has an opinion, and what works for one person may not work for you, but the more information you have to consider, the more empowered and responsible your decision will be. Remember, you make the ultimate decision.

Prepare your questions

For most interactions in healthcare, especially new provider appointments, to go as smoothly as possible, you have to come prepared. After all, there is a limited amount of time to get through much information, and you want to maximize your time, increase your efficiency, and get your questions answered as smoothly and quickly as possible.

Consider these tips for preparing for a second opinion consultation.

Organize all of your relevant medical records

This should include imaging results, test results, and previous diagnoses.

Set your provider up for success by ensuring that all your healthcare information is available for them to review before the appointment.

TIP

Make sure you bring an updated list of all medications you are taking or have recently taken. Sometimes medication side-effects can cause new symptoms to develop.

Make sure that all your documentation is easy to navigate

Prepare a summary of current events clearly and concisely. The last thing you want to be doing is flipping through stacks of papers, scrolling back and forth on your phone for pictures, or doing anything else that takes away from the time you could be conversing with your clinician about your present issues.

Keeping your information organized in a dedicated binder (if you prefer a good old-fashioned hard copy) or allowing it to be uploaded to your computer in a specific folder makes it easier for you to refer to resources and for your provider to review them.

Prepare a list of questions

These questions should be specific to your diagnosis, treatment options, and prognosis.

- Questions that have more of an administrative or operational bend to them, like the provider's communication policy, appointment scheduling, questions about cancelation policies, and more, can be answered by the doctor's office management or front desk. Write your questions down and call the doctor's office a couple of days in advance to ask those questions.
- Questions more specific to your condition, such as recommended treatment options, side-effects of treatment options, length of recovery, and confirmation or questioning of initial diagnosis, should be asked during the appointment.

By following this process, you minimize the probability of asking the wrong party-specific questions and can spend more time getting answers from the experts about things that matter most to you.

Evaluate different medical perspectives

Getting a second opinion is only half the battle. Now, you should take time to review all the information so you can determine the best plan forward.

Here are a few actions you can take to figure out what to do next:

- **Compare the second opinion to the initial diagnosis and look for any discrepancies or new information and insights.** Play a game of spot-the-difference with the information. In spot-the-difference, you are looking at two seemingly identical pictures and need to, you guessed it, spot the differences between the two. Compare the notes and information in your chart to see what is consistent in their findings and what is different:

- Did one provider highlight a treatment option that the other provider did not?
- Did one provider suggest a treatment plan that seemed more robust in comparison to the others or highlight a new possible diagnosis?
- Did one diagnosis feel more complete?
- Did one treatment plan align better with your values and goals?

» **Weigh the pros and cons of each approach.** Note the similarities and differences between your initial diagnosis and the second opinion, including each approach's positives and potential negatives. Make sure to list things like side-effects of different medications or treatment interventions, financial commitments, length of treatment, ability to complete the course of treatment, and more.

REMEMBER

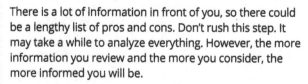

There is a lot of information in front of you, so there could be a lengthy list of pros and cons. Don't rush this step. It may take a while to analyze everything. However, the more information you review and the more you consider, the more informed you will be.

» **Identify key differences between the second opinion and the initial diagnosis and discuss these differences with a healthcare provider you trust.** The good news is that you don't have to make these decisions alone. If you have a member of your healthcare team that you trust, such as your primary care physician, talk with them about the direction you're leaning relative to the opinion that makes the most sense for you.

This person should understand your core values and goals for your health and present you with a safe space to think through your options. You might not feel comfortable with either perspective, and that's okay.

WARNING

Make sure that the decision, even if it's in collaboration with other clinicians and people you trust, is yours and one that you're comfortable with. If you have more questions or need more information about a particular approach, reach out to the provider whose plan, diagnosis, or treatment you're questioning and further the conversation. There's nothing wrong with gathering other professional opinions about your best course of action, but you make the final decision.

IN THIS CHAPTER

» Understanding what coverage gaps are

» Handling the claims process like a pro

» Resolving billing errors

» Creating a plan to address medical debt

Chapter 12 Resolving Insurance Challenges

Health insurance is undoubtedly one of the most confusing processes a patient manages. The terms are confusing, the processes seem to overlap and still don't make sense, and there is still a decent probability that the bill you receive from the insurance company will not be correct. So what do you do when you are face to face with an insurance problem and have no choice but to address it? Where do you start? Who do you ask? What are you supposed to do?

In this chapter, I dive into common insurance challenges that patients face, offer an introduction to practical solutions and insights, and equip you with introductory knowledge to overcome your insurance obstacles.

TIP

This chapter covers private insurance plans. If you are looking for specific information about Medicare, turn to Chapter 3.

Recognizing and Understanding Coverage Gaps

You would think that avoiding insurance challenges would be as simple as just having health insurance. Sure, you could understand having to deal with issues regarding the payment of your care if you didn't have insurance, but you do. Now, you're being told that your insurance is not enough or incomplete. That is the dreaded *coverage gap*.

A coverage gap is an event or a period of time in which your insurance does not fully cover certain services, treatments, or other expenses. Humor me and think about your insurance as the roof on your house. Your roof does what it needs to do, which is protect you, your loved ones, and your property from the outside elements. But, one day, a storm comes by, ripping a hole in your roof, and pouring rain rushes into your house.

The roof represents your health insurance and the hole in your roof represents any insurance coverage gaps you have. It's the part of your healthcare that's not covered by your insurance. When you have a gap in your coverage, it becomes your responsibility to finance the tests, medicines, visits, and so on.

Gaps in coverage can happen when you lose the employer-sponsored health insurance from your job, when you start a medication or treatment that's not fully covered by your primary health insurance, when your coverage lapses, or other event-specific considerations.

Although insurance coverage gaps can occur following a specific event, such as leaving or losing a job, there are ways you can better position yourself to understand what your insurance covers. The following sections discuss some ways to avoid or mitigate coverage gaps.

Regularly review your health insurance policy

Your insurance policy is your agreement between you and your health insurance company about your medical coverage. As boring and as tedious as it sounds, understanding your insurance coverage helps you avoid surprise bills. Check for changes on a regular basis. See Figure 12-1.

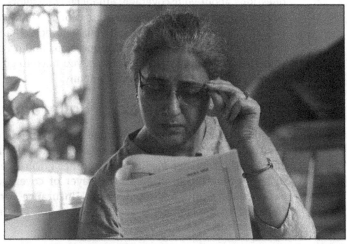

triloks/Getty Images

FIGURE 12-1: Getting a grasp on what's covered and what's not can be difficult!

If you know that you will be undergoing a specific kind of treatment or starting a new medication, call your insurance company and ask if that intervention is covered and to what extent.

TIP

If you have more than one insurance carrier, review all of them and make sure you understand how they overlap and who pays for what (also called *coordination of benefits*).

Consider how significant life changes affect your coverage needs

For example, if you are laid off from your job and no longer eligible for your employee health plan, reach out to your human resources representative or other relevant stakeholder to learn more about enrollment to COBRA, which allows you to continue your employee health plan benefits for a temporary, specified amount of time (usually 18 months). Life events like getting married or the death of a spouse or person whose healthcare plan you are on can also affect your coverage.

Ask your insurance company

Be sure to reach out to your insurance company when you have questions about your coverage. Financial counselors, medical bill advocates, and other healthcare professionals that help you navigate the financial components of your healthcare journey may be able to help you with a number of questions and processes about your insurance. However, sometimes you have to go right to the source and talk to the insurance company.

Consider adding extra coverage

To make your insurance coverage more complete, consider additional support. Private insurance can be expensive, so if you qualify, consider Medicaid or another government program to help provide you an additional layer of coverage. Medicare patients may consider supplemental insurance for their plan (referred to as Medigap). See Chapter 3 for lots more about Medicare and Medicaid.

Hire a patient advocate

Some patient advocates specialize in insurance navigation and medical financial support.

Hiring an expert patient advocate who understands how to work with insurance companies could be helpful. They can suggest ways to improve the resiliency of your insurance coverage, help dispute medical bills, and more. If you've been recently diagnosed with an illness that requires you to complete an increased number of treatments or start a new medication, a patient advocate can help make sure you can resiliently navigate any insurance hurdles.

Navigating the Claims Process

When you need a treatment or service, such as a medical procedure, your healthcare provider submits an insurance claim to your insurance company requesting payment for the service they provided. Generally, you work with your healthcare provider to receive a service and the claim is filed on your behalf.

You can submit the claim, or your provider can do it. The *claim* is a formal bill (like an invoice) that outlines information, like your diagnosis (the diagnosis code), the date of service, the procedure code of the medical intervention, and more. From there, your insurance company makes sure all the information on the claim is correct and compares it to your plan, so they can pay for what is covered and bill you for what is not.

If your claim is approved, the insurance pays for the services. If it's denied, you're usually sent an explanation of benefits that shows the breakdown of what they paid for and what they did not. You may be stuck with the bill.

To set yourself up for success and to increase the probability of your claim being approved, keep these tips in mind:

- **Make sure you understand what your insurance policy says about cover treatments, procedures, and more.** Be familiar with what is excluded, what is allowed, and to what limits.
- **When you can, stay in network.** Staying *in-network* means utilizing the services of healthcare providers that belong to hospitals and clinics that have agreed to work with your insurance company. If you get treatment from providers outside of your network, you're out of pocket fees might be relatively high.
- **Don't take no for an answer.** If your claim is denied, you have the right to appeal it. Reach out to your insurance company to understand why it was denied, what other documentation might be needed to support a successful appeal, and the time frame in which you need to take action. Ask for an explanation of benefits.
- **Make sure that the supporting documentation and clinical information is correct and complete.** That means everything from the spelling of your name, to the date the service was performed, and even how it was billed by medical billers. Errors can result in denied claims.
- **Heed the deadlines for submitting claims and appeals.** If they give you 60 days, that means 60 days. Don't risk your claims being automatically thrown out because of a time management issue.
- **Keep tabs on your claim.** As awesome and individual as you are, you are one of maybe millions of claims that need to be processed by the insurance company. If you receive

correspondence that you're supposed to hear back regarding the status of a claim within a certain time frame and you don't hear back, ask for an update.

Billing Errors! Where to Start and Who to Talk To

Everyone understands that mistakes happen. However, it's not so easy to graciously forgive a billing error, especially if the charges are wildly incorrect, inflated, or just plain unsubstantiated. Even the most prestigious health systems turn out bills for services that are incorrect to patients, and it happens more often than you think.

REMEMBER

The number one cause of billing errors is inaccurate patient information. Make sure you keep your information up to date and double-check all those forms you sign to ensure that this doesn't happen to you!

Dealing with these issues can be frustrating and extremely time-consuming. On the bright side, there are ways to resolve them.

TIP

Above all, consider the advice of the impactful, late-great patient advocate Marshall Allen, who coined the patient call to action, "Never pay the first bill!"

If your bill is incorrect but you pay it anyway, you might not get that money back. Make that what you're being asked to pay is correct, after the proper entities, such as your insurance plan, have paid their part.

Show the proof!

Make sure that you provide all copies of bills, receipts, and other information that support your claim that you have been improperly billed. Insurance companies must be able to review proof of documentation that shows they made an error. You might need to play detective when it comes to your medical bills.

TIP

Some billing discrepancies can be found in the comparison between the bill you received and the explanation of benefits from the insurance company. If you don't recognize a charge or a service name, highlight it on the bill and put it aside as you build your case.

Contact your hospital's billing department

Let them know that you believe you've identified a discrepancy and would like an itemized bill, or a broken down list of services, treatments, and prices. Then make sure that list matches the care you actually received.

Put your concerns in writing

If you are unable to work through the billing discrepancies by working with your hospital finance department and the insurance company, you can formally submit a dispute. Make sure all that proof that you gathered goes along with it.

REMEMBER

You get more bees with honey than you do with vinegar. Sometimes billing errors can be resolved with a few calls to the appropriate financial department. Speak to people regarding your bill with respect, even though you may be fuming on the inside.

Make sure that you are being professional and polite to the agents that are trying to help you. Professional and polite doesn't mean being a pushover, so don't dismiss the issue to be perceived as an agreeable person The facts are the facts — the bill is wrong — and you are looking for assistance in correcting the issue.

TIP

It's best to get a real person on the phone instead of a voicemail box. Keep calling back to make this happen.

Tackling Medical Debt

Navigating the management of your healthcare is hard enough, but adding the overwhelming concern and burden of medical bills, coverage plans with limitations, and high deductibles to the scenario (all under the umbrella term of medical debt) can make the healthcare experience a real nightmare.

In countries that do not have national health coverage, like the United States, medical debt can essentially break the financial well-being of a patient.

This section covers some tips and techniques for managing medical debt.

Review the accuracy of the bills

You can nip unnecessary and inflated costs in the bud by taking the time to make sure that the bills you receive are accurate and cover only the services, treatments, and medications you've actually been administered. If your bill is wrong and you don't call it out and have it fixed, that incorrect balance could become a part of your financial obligation.

If you don't owe it, take the appropriate actions to prove it and get it wiped from your account.

Hold your insurance company accountable

Make sure you are familiar with the contract or policy of your insurance plan so that you know what your insurance company is supposed to pay, how much, when, and to what extent. If you receive bills for services that should be covered by your insurance, follow the appropriate claims processes to ensure that they're paid by the appropriate party, which in this case is not you.

REMEMBER

Things like your co-pays, payments toward your deductible, and other factors are likely your responsibility, per the stipulations of your insurance policy.

Look into hospital and patient assistance programs

Even if you've made the appropriate efforts to ensure that you're only paying for what you should be paying for, the out of pocket expense can still be overwhelming.

It never hurts to ask about financial assistance programs that your hospital or other community resources have and see if you qualify. If you meet the criteria for the program, you can utilize the benefits and help combat the amount of money you have to pay yourself.

TIP

Financial assistance programs and patient assistance programs may exist outside of your health system, such as through patient advocacy organizations and charity funds. If you're a veteran, be sure to consider your VA benefits. Chapter 3 covers the VA health insurance.

Some pharmaceutical company have financial assistance programs to help patients afford certain medications they offer. You can ask your local pharmacist or your provider about this or check the pharmaceutical company's website for information.

Consider setting up a payment plan

You can do this with the billing department. Just because you don't pay down the debt doesn't mean it goes away. Making even small, incremental payments toward this debt may help manage expectations. They may be less likely to send your medical debt to a collection agency if you continue to pay it down in-house. If your ability to pay your previously agreed upon amount or time frame changes, reach out to the department and see how it can be adjusted to better suit your current state.

TIP

If medical debt collectors reach out to you demanding payment, remember that you have rights. The Fair Debt Collection Practices Act (`www.ftc.gov/legal-library/browse/rules/fair-debt-collection-practices-act-text`) gives you the right to dispute a debt within 30 days of a debt collector contacting you. The collection agency should also be able to prove that you owe the debt they are attempting to collect. Research your options, including settlements and filing bankruptcy, with finance professionals.

Reach out when you need help navigating your options

Consider working with a financial advisor, patient advocate, or another reputable professional for advice on how to make your medical debt less daunting.

IN THIS CHAPTER

» Planning for the evolving health needs of chronic conditions

» Understanding the difference among the long-term care options

» Managing chronic conditions at work

Chapter 13 Navigating Chronic Conditions and Long-Term Care

Chronic health conditions, such as diabetes, hypertension, and cancer, can require long-term management and potentially alter aspects of a person's daily life. This chapter explores chronic and long-term conditions, explains how to discuss evolving needs with the care team, and covers different care options — such as assisted living and skilled nursing facilities. You'll also find guidance on other factors to consider when planning for ongoing healthcare needs, whether it's yours or a loved one's.

Understanding Chronic Health Conditions

Long-term or chronic health conditions require continuous management over a long period, possibly over a lifetime. Managing these conditions can involve taking medication, making lifestyle adjustments, visiting the clinician frequently, and handling persistent pain and symptoms. The bright side? People living with chronic conditions can lead fulfilling lives, especially when they maintain regular care, collaborate with their healthcare providers to focus on their quality of life, and establish attainable management goals for their condition.

If you've been diagnosed with a chronic condition — for example, diabetes, arthritis, Crohn's disease, fibromyalgia, cancer, asthma, or GERD — it's helpful to familiarize yourself with key terms related to chronic care. Many conditions have "episodic" symptoms, which come and go. Unlike an infection or injury that can heal completely, chronic conditions generally don't go away in the same way.

Chronic conditions typically last longer than three months and are not contagious. Appropriate support, along with self-care practices, enable many patients with chronic conditions to live fulfilling lives. To make the most of your diagnosis, you need to understand which body systems the condition affects so you can manage the condition over time.

Planning for Long-Term Care Needs

Chronic illnesses and disabilities are often part of a lifelong journey, requiring regular assessment, a proactive mindset, and planning. By knowing your condition's present state and how it may progress over time, you can feel empowered to live a life centered around your values and goals while prioritizing your health.

Here are a few steps to help you approach this journey with confidence and resilience:

» **Seek continuous evaluation and open dialogue.**

  Chronic conditions evolve, which makes regular consultation with your healthcare team essential. Work closely with your care team to assess your current needs and plan for potential future challenges. Your age, lifestyle, and overall health might impact how your condition progresses. Don't think of this planning as a negative look into the future; instead, consider it as building a roadmap that helps you thrive.

» **Define personal priorities and values.**

Maybe maintaining independence is important to you. Communicating this to your healthcare team and support network ensures they can assist you in preserving your independence for as long as possible, even as your condition changes.

» **Advocate to your support network.**

Your support team — family, friends, and healthcare providers — can offer valuable perspectives. Work together to identify realistic plans and solutions for the future, ensuring that your care aligns with your values and lifestyle goals.

» **Plan for key milestones with purpose (and checklists).** Breaking down the process into steps can help make long-term planning more manageable.

Table 13-1 shows a sample checklist to get you started.

TIP

When the unexpected happens, like a significant change in your health status, a fall, or another significant consideration, take the time to understand how that change could affect your long-term plan.

» **Be flexible and adaptive.**

As your circumstances and priorities shift, keep your planning flexible. Routine reviews help you remain active and forward-thinking in your healthcare management.

TABLE 13-1 Sample Checklist

Action	Description
Create a care binder	A binder or digital file that includes medical records, emergency contacts, medication lists, and important care instructions. This binder serves as a "go-to" resource for you and your support team. This makes it easier to be prepared to meet with different clinicians, transition between inpatient and outpatient support, and many other factors.
Review your care plans regularly	Schedule annual or semi-annual check-ins with your care team to review your health, discuss any changes, and update your care plan.
Plan for the future	Think about potential future adjustments, such as mobility aids, home modifications, or accessible living arrangements, and discuss them with your care team.

By planning, you're setting up a foundation for a life that aligns with your values and goals, from the get-go, even as you navigate the challenges of a chronic condition. Remember, your care journey is about not only surviving, but about thriving in a way that honors what's most important to you.

Understanding Your Care Options

Contrary to popular belief, there are big differences between the care options currently available in the United States. This section contains a quick overview of common options to help you get the basics and ask the right questions.

In-home care versus home healthcare

In-home care offers the least disruption to your current, everyday life, letting you stay in the comfort of your own home while getting assistance with daily tasks like preparing meals, doing laundry, or bathing. This assistance is not medical care. Patients recovering from surgery and medically cleared for discharge may find the support helpful with such an option. It's a flexible option that can happen around your own schedule, but often comes without out-of-pocket costs, as many insurance plans don't cover it. Work with your care team, insurance provider, and the leadership of in-home care agencies tell get a clear financial picture for your situation.

TIP

You can ask for free assessments from home care agencies to get a better understanding of what your insurance covers, what the agency services offer, and whether they are a good fit — all without having to make a financial obligation.

WARNING

Understanding the distinction between in-home care and home healthcare is crucial for avoiding confusion and unforeseen expenses:

- **In-home care** focuses on non-medical help, such as assistance tasks like cooking, cleaning, and other daily activities. This empowers people to maintain independence in their home. This type of care is non-medical, and it usually isn't covered by standard health insurance and might necessitate out-of-pocket payments or coverage through long-term care insurance.

TIP

As of the writing of this book, Medicaid may cover in-home care. Reach out to your Medicaid provider for more information about eligibility.

» **Home healthcare** aims to provide medical support, including services like wound care, medication management, physical therapy, and more, delivered by licensed professionals such as nurses and therapists. Typically, health insurance, Medicare, or Medicaid covers this kind of care when your clinician prescribes it and you meet the eligibility criteria.

Understanding the differences between these options can help you make informed decisions about the care you need while effectively managing costs. See Chapter 3 for more about Medicare, Medicaid, and other types of insurance.

Adult day care

Adult day care is a helpful resource for people who mostly live independently. Adult day care services provide daytime supervision and activities and social engagements. They can provide increased safety in a supervised environment for some patients, as well as potentially allowing support family and caregivers an opportunity to rest, work, and do other things that they need to do knowing that the patient is in a safe environment.

Adult day care is sometimes covered by insurance like Medicaid or long-term care insurance, depending on where you live. (If you have limited financial resources, you may be eligible for Medicaid waiver programs. This can be a great fit for people who live with family but need some structure during the day.)

TIP

Medicaid waivers give patients with certain conditions and disabilities the ability to receive certain care in other settings, like in their community or home, as opposed to just in a hospital or long-term care facility. Your state manages this program, so check with your State Department of Medicaid for eligibility requirements, services covered, and more.

TIP

There are several kinds of adult day care models. Some focus on social stimulation (like recreational activities) and don't have medical supervision, while others support patients with specific conditions, like Alzheimer's.

Assisted living facilities

Assisted living offers moderate support. It's ideal for people who don't need constant medical monitoring but do need some help with activities of daily living (ADLs). Facilities often offer private or semi-private living spaces, meal support, and amenities to help residents maintain independence. The support provided here is centered on grooming, help to the bathroom, and getting dressed — not on providing intense medical care. Some facilities may also provide memory care for those with dementia.

At the time of writing this book, Medicare generally doesn't cover assisted living facilities. Many residents pay out of pocket, but check with your insurance for potential coverage or for options to help absorb the cost. See Figure 13-1.

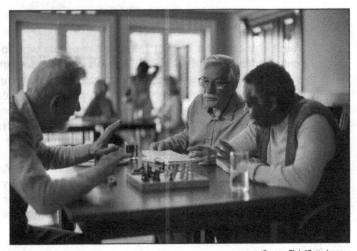

Drazen Zigic/Getty Images

FIGURE 13-1: Assisted living facilities can provide comfort, everyday task support, and camaraderie to elderly loved ones.

FIND ONLINE

If you are a U.S. veteran (or married to one), you may be entitled to additional support that can help you pay for assistant living, like the Veterans Aid and Attendance Benefit. Your eligibility depends on your service specifics and financial need. See Chapter 3 or the U.S Department of Veterans Affairs Guide to Long-Term Care (`www.va.gov/geriatrics`) for more information about VA health insurance.

Memory care facilities

These specialized environments cater to individuals with memory challenges and cognitive impairments, ensuring a secure setting that emphasizes safety and structure. The staff has specialized training to care for patients with cognitive impairments like Alzheimer's or dementia. Other facilities may have the capacity to support Alzheimer patients and other patients with memory challenges, but the care may be more general compared to specialized memory care.

While these facilities generally come with higher costs than regular assisted living, do your research so that you get a clear picture of the financial investment.

Make sure you understand which aspects of memory care are covered by your insurance. For example, Medicare may cover some, but not all, of memory care costs. Health insurance companies can cover all, none, or a percentage of services, so be sure to determine what part of the tab they pick up, if any.

TIP

Always take a tour of any facility you are considering. To learn more about a care facility, ask for the Special Care Unit Disclosure during your tour. This form can help you make the best decision about the facility based on transparent information on topics that are important to you and the patient.

Skilled nursing facilities (SNFs)

Skilled nursing facilities (often called nursing homes or SNFs and pronounced "sniffs"), provide 24/7 care to patients who need continuous medical care or rehabilitation. Patients with complex health conditions that need regular medication attention can benefit from this option.

Many patients and their families express serious worries about the safety or quality of nursing homes. Finding facilities that meet your needs, offer safe care, and don't have long waiting lists can be difficult. Do your homework up front. Be sure to check in with your loved one regularly to make sure that:

- » They feel safe.
- » Their personal care and medical care needs are being met.
- » Their health is not deteriorating beyond expectations of the normal aging process.

The Center for Medicare and Medicaid Services (CMS) has a skilled nursing facility checklist that you can use to help you compare skilled nursing facilities before your select one. Check it out at `medicare.gov`.

TIP

Consider choosing a Continuing Care Retirement Community (CCRC) if you want to access multiple care levels in one facility. CCRC residents can access different support levels through multiple care options in one place, as their needs change (like moving from memory care to a SNF). Although CCRCs come with considerable out-of-pocket costs, they may be a great investment for those who want to "age in place."

Independent living communities

Independent living communities are housing options for older people who want to remain independent and enjoy the company of community.

Consider independent living communities if you are overall healthy, active, and need minimal assistance. These facilities do not provide medical support for residents, although staff may be available in the event of an emergency. Residents often pay a flat fee that may include meals, amenity access, and more.

Coverages like Medicare and Medicaid don't cover independent senior living, but may cover medical services received at these facilities. Check with your insurance company to understand your cost-sharing.

FIND ONLINE

For patients with disabilities, Centers for Independent Living (CILs) can be a phenomenal resource to get information on how to transition from facilities, like nursing homes, into the community to live independently, provide peer support, and more. CILs are funded by the state but run by other people with disabilities. Find a CIL near you on the National Council on Independent Living website (`https://ncil.org/about/find-your-cil-list`).

While this isn't an exhaustive list of every possible long-term care option, it highlights some of the key paths worth exploring. Treat this as a starting point for meaningful discussions with your care team as you chart the best course ahead — whether it's for yourself or a loved one. Your choices are deeply personal, so take this opportunity to align the care pathway with what's truly important to you and your family.

TIP

If you don't know which long term care option works for you, ask your provider. You can also ask for a geriatric care assessment (or comprehensive geriatric assessment) to evaluate aspects like physical health and functional ability. This gives data to support further decision making.

Managing Changes to Your Care Options

Living with a chronic condition means being ready for change. Your care plan isn't set in stone — it needs to evolve just like your needs do. What works well today might not be the best tomorrow.

- Remain flexible and keep track of your needs to make timely adjustments.
- Having open, honest conversations with your healthcare team is crucial.
- As new symptoms or challenges arise, let them guide you in tweaking your care plan. This ongoing dialogue ensures your care evolves with you.

When caring for someone else, make routine check-ins a priority. These are opportunities to review what's effective, tackle any new issues, and discover potential treatments that might benefit you moving forward. Staying informed helps the care plan stay relevant, enabling the loved one to live their best life.

Why adjusting care settings is important

Adjusting care settings as health needs change is vital for preserving your safety, freedom, and quality of life as your health evolves — whether due to aging, a chronic condition progressing, or unexpected changes — the support you require may shift, necessitating a new environment.

Deliberate adjustments can increase safety and help avert accidents, mainly as physical and cognitive transformations occur. Engage in open, forward-thinking dialogue with your healthcare team and your loved ones.

Preparing for smooth(er) care transitions

When it's time to think about changing the level of care, planning ahead can make things a lot easier. You want to avoid that "scramble mode" if something suddenly changes. Here's a quick guide to help you or your loved one adjust more smoothly:

TIP

- **Plan early, stress less.**

  Regularly check in with your healthcare team to address your needs early on, so decisions aren't rushed in a crisis. Early planning allows you to organize finances, understand insurance, and explore your options thoroughly.

  Create a short list of facilities in the geographically desired area to use as the healthcare journey progresses. Facilities should have safe staffing to residents ratios, adequate licensure protocol for continuous staff training, reasonable staff turnover rates, strict protocols for resident safety and infection prevention, and more. You can revisit this list depending on finances, the type of care that's needed, preferences, and more. Start gathering information about these facilities by calling them and asking questions and then visiting your top five. Modify your top contenders given wait lists and other factors that might affect move-in.

- **Anticipate when a change is needed.**

  Talk with your support network to identify which signs mean it's time for a new care setting. For example, are falls becoming more frequent? Is hygiene a struggle? Spotting these changes early can help you stay on top of things before they become too overwhelming.

- **Prepare for the emotional impact.**

  The transition into a new place is a big change, especially if you've lived somewhere for a long time. College students feel the stress when they move out of their parent's place to the dorms for the first time. Even empty-nesters feel it when moving from the larger house they raised their family to a smaller place — it's exciting, but can also feel weird. Working with a counselor or mental health professional can help ease the transition.

» **Build a solid support team.**

If you live far away or cannot otherwise manage your loved one's care, choose a trusted person like a family member or friend or hire a professional patient advocate to take on this responsibility. They can keep you in the loop and help manage the process.

TIP

If you appoint a trusted friend or someone else to help manage the process with you, make sure the patient is involved in that dynamic and that the proper legal paperwork is filed so they can access the medical records or be included in conversations about the patient's health.

» **Respect individual goals and wishes.**

Everyone has preferences. Some people want to live independently, while others may prefer community living. Talk with the care team to explore options that respect these goals — even if compromise is needed.

» **Do your homework and visit facilities!**

Don't just rely on websites or brochures — visit the facilities. Bring someone you trust, ask all the questions you want, and pay attention to how it feels. Trust your gut! Sometimes you can learn a lot just by seeing how staff interact. Is the place clean? Do the other residents look happy? Is the staff attentive? By being at the facilities in person, you may have the opportunity to talk to some of the residents and learn more about their experience.

TIP

It may sound trivial, but things like the quality of the food could be a big seller, or a big drawback. If you're going to live someplace that's going to provide you a number of meals a day, you probably want to enjoy them. Make a point to look around the cafeteria, or even have lunch there to get the real scoop. For patients with specific dietary needs and management of their care, being knowledgeable of how prospective facilities and care options address these is important.

» **Make the move gradual (where possible).**

Moving can feel like a big leap. To avoid "new place shock," try to make the space feel familiar. Bring favorite items, set up routines, and work with professionals on ways to ease into the new environment.

» **Create a good old-fashioned pro and cons list.**

When there are so many options, organizing info can help a lot. Make a list of pros and cons or a comparison chart, including things like costs, location, services, accommodations, and how the place felt on the tour. Seeing everything in one spot makes decision-making way easier. Make sure to add pros and cons that are not just logistically important but important to you to the list as well. May you have a pet that you want to move with you. Be sure to note the facilities that are pet-friendly.

» **Embrace the emotional ups and downs.**

Change can be a mix of excitement and nerves. Whether it's moving to a smaller place or to a new care setting, expect a range of emotions. Take time to process these feelings and don't hesitate to use support resources to help.

» **Ask all the questions and lean on experts.**

No question is too small! Be open about your concerns and use the experience of healthcare pros to help you make the best decision. Their guidance helps eliminate guesswork from situations that may initially seem overwhelming.

With thoughtful planning, active questioning, and taking things step-by-step, you can transition to a new care setting smoothly and without the hassle of hasty, last-minute choices.

Financial Considerations for Long-Term Care

Affording long-term care isn't like managing costs for regular doctor visits. While routine healthcare usually involves insurance coverage and some out-of-pocket expenses, planning for long-term care requires a unique financial approach. Comprehensive financial planning grants you more flexibility in choosing the kind of support you desire as your needs evolve.

This section is a snapshot of the main avenues people use to navigate long-term care costs — savings, financial assets, insurance, and government programs — and some pointers on how to get started.

» **Insurance probably won't cover all aspects of long-term care, so you may be responsible for significant out-of-pocket expenses.** Work with financial advisors or counselors to create a realistic budget and identify ways to earmark funds specifically for these needs. Additionally, consulting with legal professionals is beneficial to review any long-term care contracts and ensure financial protection in case of any changes with your chosen facility, such as a loss of accreditation.

» **Start building your savings now.** Review your current assets, cash flow, and financial factors, and set aside funds for future care requirements.

» **Consider long-term care insurance as an option.** Policies are generally either traditional, focusing solely on long-term care, or hybrid, which may include extras like death benefits.

FIND ONLINE

Long-term care insurance information is also accessible through resources like `longtermcare.gov`, which offers information on selecting an agent or financial planner, and details on state programs.

» **Understanding government programs like Medicaid and Medicare is vital in the long-term care framework.** Medicaid often supports long-term care services but only for those who qualify and to certain limits. Dependable sources, such as the Centers for Medicare and Medicaid Services (CMS), can provide current information on coverage and duration.

TIP

While Medicare does not usually cover long-term care expenses, it may provide limited short-term skilled nursing facility (SNF) coverage following hospital stays for up to 100 days. Medicare might also cover certain home healthcare services (not to be confused with in-home care) on a limited basis, if deemed medically necessary. Medicare typically does not cover assisted living or long-term; however, there can be some exceptions based on specific qualifying criteria.

Medicaid, on the other hand, is often accessible to patients with limited income or assets and can offer more substantial long-term care coverage, including nursing home support and, in some cases, assisted living support. Since Medicaid eligibility is based on financial need, it can be more accessible for individuals who meet these income criteria.

These general guidelines can help set expectations, but a thorough review of your individual coverage will provide a more accurate understanding. See Chapter 3 as well.

TIP

As you explore the care options, request a cost breakdown for services like in-home care versus assisted living to be clear on potential out-of-pocket costs. You can also ask your employer about any available pension benefits, long-term care programs, or discounts.

While navigating long-term care finances might seem daunting, working with patient advocates and financial professionals can clarify the process and ensure informed decision-making. Planning ahead and grasping your options means you'll be better prepared to prioritize your care needs over time.

Legal Aspects of Long-Term Care

Understanding the legal considerations is essential when you explore long-term care options. Be sure you understand issues like payment responsibilities, decision-making processes regarding changing care levels, and the scope of services provided.

Establishing legal protections before any potential care transition is vital. This includes setting up healthcare powers of attorney, living wills, and other advance directives to outline your care preferences clearly. These documents might designate someone to decide on your behalf if you cannot specify your wishes regarding life-sustaining treatments. Chapter 18 delves deeper into these considerations.

TIP

Engage in these discussions sooner rather than later. Although it might feel difficult, documenting your preferences now can ensure they are respected should you be unable to communicate them later. For further assistance, reach out to your care team for resources or recommendations for professionals who can aid in these critical conversations and documentation.

Involving Family and Caregivers in Decision Making

Family, in whatever way you define it, along with close friends and caregivers, can play a crucial role in helping you make decisions about your current and future care. You have the right to involve your support network in your healthcare journey in your healthcare decisions to whatever extent you feel comfortable.

Have open conversations with those you trust about:

- Your goals for care
- The support you'll appreciate as your needs evolve
- The roles you envision for your loved ones for support

While these conversations aren't always easy, starting with an update about your care can open the door. For instance, if you're managing a chronic condition, you might share with your loved ones that while you're handling it well now, the support you need may change over time.

Inviting their thoughts and feelings into this dialogue can establish a shared understanding. You should not feel compelled to accept someone else's opinion simply because of their connection to you — everyone has a unique perspective.

Your friends and family members might take turns sharing caregiving duties, which includes managing household activities and going with you to medical visits. Caregiving has an emotional and physical impact on our loved ones — make it a habit to check in with one another.

Create safe spaces to discuss not only updates on your health but also how everyone is feeling about the situation. Sometimes, patients may feel guilty about relying on loved ones, yet often family and friends want to be there for you in every way possible. See Figure 13-2.

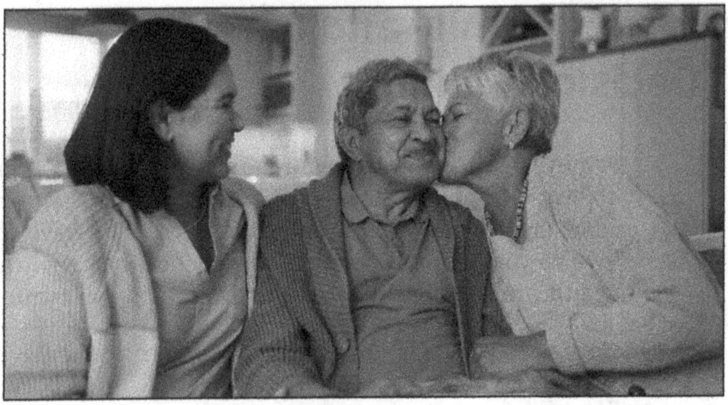

Jacob Wackerhausen/Getty Images

FIGURE 13-2: In the best scenarios, making decisions together about long-term care can bring family together.

As a group, work together to make choices that feel right for you while supporting the mental health and well-being of everyone involved. Involving a mental health professional in this process can also be invaluable in navigating complex feelings and maintaining a healthy balance in these supportive relationships.

Managing Chronic Health Conditions in the Workplace

Your ability to work can be substantially affected by chronic conditions. As your condition changes, it can affect your physical abilities, energy levels, focus, and productivity.

Here are key points to consider when managing chronic conditions in the workplace:

» **Know your rights for workplace accommodations.**

Understanding your rights as an employee is key to managing your work responsibilities and your health needs. Under the Americans with Disabilities Act (ADA), employers must provide reasonable accommodations for employees with chronic conditions. Reasonable accommodations could include flexible hours, ergonomic equipment, and remote work options. Consult with your HR representative and clinical care team to begin the process of requesting accommodations. See Figure 13-3.

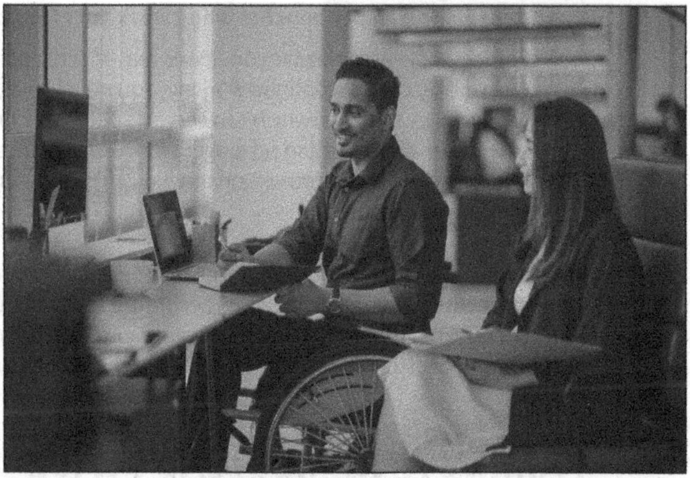

Edwin Tan / iStockphoto

FIGURE 13-3: Employers must provide reasonable accommodations for employees with disabilities.

- **Explore sick leave and disability options.**

  The Family and Medical Leave Act (FMLA; see the sidebar) and other health-related leave policies could make you eligible for leave time. If your condition affects your work capacity temporarily or permanently, you may be able to access short-term or long-term disability benefits. Consult with HR and your healthcare team confidentially to learn how to apply for and manage your benefits.

- **Prioritize your health and well-being at work.**

  Managing a chronic condition while working is a balancing act, so prioritize your health. Take breaks when you're able. Remember, putting your health first is a necessity — not an option.

- **Develop a work-life balance that fits your needs.**

  Collaborate with your HR department and supervisor to develop a workplace atmosphere that supports your productivity and focuses on your well-being. This collaboration may lead to redefining your work hours, reducing stress, or arranging your workspace to better meet your physical requirements. If your current department can't support changes to work, explore other positions what may align better.

» **Consider disability benefits when work isn't feasible.**

Some people with chronic conditions may reach a point where they cannot continue working. You may be eligible for disability benefits, which can serve as necessary financial assistance when you can no longer work. Explore these options with trusted professionals who can guide you through the process.

By staying informed about your rights, understanding workplace resources, and openly discussing accommodations that support your current healthcare journey with your care team, you can prioritize your health while managing a chronic condition at work.

FAMILY AND MEDICAL LEAVE ACT (FMLA)

The Family and Medical Leave Act (FMLA) ensures that eligible workers keep their employment while taking up to 12 weeks per year of unpaid time off. This can be for family reasons, such as caring for a sick child, parent, or spouse, and for medical needs, such as serious health conditions. Military family leave provisions also exist under FMLA. Eligible employees can use leave intermittently or all at once. To become eligible for FMLA protection, employees need to fulfill certain work conditions and employer size requirements.

Visit the U.S. Department of Labor website (`https://www.dol.gov/agencies/whd/fmla/faq#14`) for more information.

IN THIS CHAPTER

» Recognizing and combating healthcare acquired infections (HAIs)

» Taking responsibility for your personal safety

» Preventing falls and fall-related injuries

Chapter 14 Protecting Yourself Against Harm

In addition to caring for you and making you well, the reality of hospitals and care centers is that being in such a setting can expose you to unanticipated risks. This includes the possibility of contracting infections, experiencing falls that could lead to serious injuries, and facing other unforeseen health complications. This chapter explores these risks of healthcare environments.

Armed with this information, you can be your own advocate. Engaging in meaningful discussions with your healthcare team can help protect you from harm while you seek care.

Recognizing HAIs

HAIs, also known as *hospital-acquired infections* or *healthcare-associated infections*, are infections you can pick up during a hospital stay or while interacting with the healthcare system. These infections aren't the same as the ones you might catch in everyday life or in your community, like the flu, a cold, or strep throat, because they often have more serious complications to your health, spread differently, and need to be treated and prevented more aggressively.

There are many kinds of HAIs. Examples include the following (see Figure 14-1):

- **SSIs (surgical site infections):** These can occur when the part of your body where your surgeon made the incision, or the surgical site, becomes infected. The infection can come from an unsterile surgical instrument like a scalpel or clamp, being used during your surgery. These can lead to serious infections like staph infections or sepsis, increased pain, and more.
- **CAUTI (catheter-associated urinary tract infections):** The most common HAIs that occurs when bacteria or other pathogens travel into the urinary tract by way of a catheter. Left untreated, they can cause discomfort for the patient, bladder infections, and other more serious infections.
- **C. diff (clostridioides difficile) infections:** A particularly virulent infection that doesn't respond well to common antibiotics and can be very difficult to treat. Even though almost every patient could be at risk for C. diff, certain populations, like patients over 65 patients or those with compromised immune systems, are often at higher risk.
- **MRSA (methicillin-resistant staphylococcus aureus):** Another potentially aggressive, contagious infection caused by an antibiotic-resistant bacterium that can spread by contact with a contaminated surface or with someone who has been infected.
- **CLABSIs (central line-associated bloodstream infections):** Infection caused by harmful bacteria entering the bloodstream through a catheter placed in large veins like the jugular on your neck. These are worrisome because they can lead to blood poisoning and organ failure in severe cases.

These aren't the only HAIs out there, but they're some of the most common. Working with your healthcare team to spot early symptoms, like a fever or new pain/swelling (especially around a surgical area), is the key to catching and treating these infections fast.

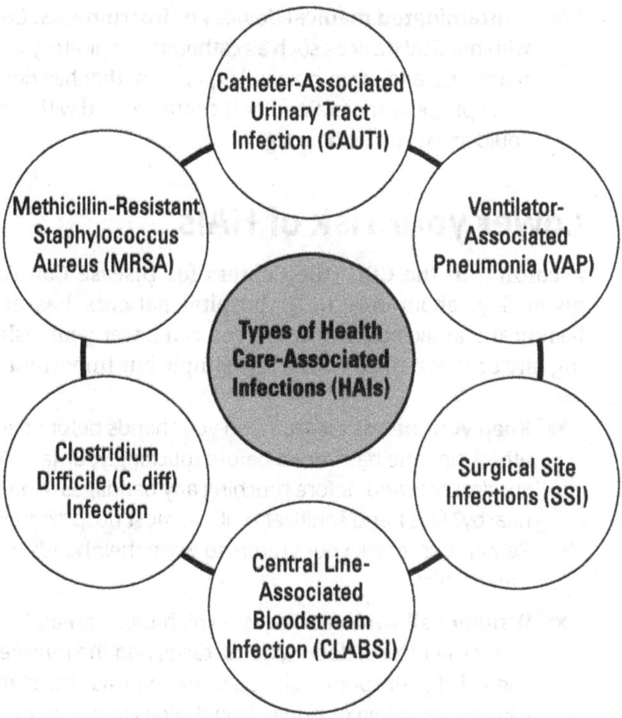

FIGURE 14-1: Common hospital-acquired infections.

How do HAIs spread?

Depending on the type, HAIs can spread in different ways, including by:

- **Touching contaminated surfaces:** From surfaces like bed rails, doorknobs, and call buttons. Germs and other pathogens pass from surfaces to hands and other body parts.
- **Air and droplets:** Through the air, especially in shared spaces. A cough or sneeze can send particles in the air for others to inhale.
- **Personal contact:** Bacteria, fungi, and viruses can spread through person-to-person contact. This includes unclean hands.

- **Contaminated medical devices or instruments:** Contact with medical devices such as catheters, respiratory machines, and other hospital equipment that has not been properly maintained or is contaminated with bacteria could leave you with an HAI.

Lower your risk of HAIs

According to the CDC (the Centers for Disease Control), on any given day, about one in 31 hospital patients has at least one healthcare-associated infection. You can lower your risk of acquiring any of these HAIs with a few simple but important processes:

- **Keep your hands clean:** Wash your hands before eating, after using the bathroom, before touching your face or surgical site, and before touching any bandages. No sink nearby? Use hand sanitizer — it's in most hospital rooms! Remember to ask your visitors to wash their hands to when they stop in.
- **Disinfect all surfaces:** Focus on high-touch areas, like bed rails, call buttons, door handles, toilet, and the remote control. If your room feels less than clean, ask the staff to wipe things down or bring alcohol wipes to give it an extra clean. They may even reclean it for you.
- **Ask questions about cleaning plans and protocols:** If you have central line or catheter or are using another medical device that stays in your body for long periods of time, ask your care team how frequently it needs to be changed or maintained.
- **Keep your eyes peeled:** Notice heavy dust on the bed rails, a moldy smell in the bathroom, or overflowing biohazard waste bins? These might be signs that the space is not being cleaned as frequently and thoroughly as it should be. If you don't feel like your space is clean, let your team know ASAP.
- **Stay up to date on your vaccines:** Illnesses, like the flu, compromise your immune system and make you more susceptible to other viruses and infections. Ask your clinician about vaccinations.
- **Be antibiotics aware:** Some bacteria that cause HAIs, like MRSA, are antibiotic resistant — the bacteria defends itself from the antibiotics you take to wipe it out. Under the

supervision of your individual care team, be sure to use antibiotics only when you need them and not "just because."

» **Keep your care team accountable:** If someone (a nurse, doctor, or anyone else) comes in to treat you and skips the hand sanitizer or sink, don't be shy — ask them to wash or sanitize their hands. Full transparency, this can be awkward, especially if the person responds that they cleaned them before they came in. However, most healthcare staff will happily do it again in front of you to give you peace-of-mind.

If you want to go the extra mile, bring your own wipes or use the ones at the hospital (be careful with these — they are strong and may require you use gloves) and wipe things over once again.

FIND ONLINE

You can learn more from reliable sources like the CDC (`cdc.gov/healthcare-associated-infections`), the World Health Organization (`https://who.int`), and the Joint Commission (`www.jointcommission.org`). They have detailed information on preventing infections in hospitals.

Steady Steps: Preventing Falls and Fall-Related Injuries

While it's true that older adults face a higher risk of falls and injuries related to them, the truth is, anyone can fall. If you are recovering from surgery, navigating mobility challenges, or just slip unexpectedly, falling can be painful and disrupt your recovery. The section discusses how to prevent them.

Know your risk

Ask your doctors and nurses whether you're at higher risk for falls. Patients with mobility challenges or who use mobility aids, like walkers and rollators, those recovering from surgery, or those managing other health conditions may be more prone to falls.

TIP

Make sure those involved in your care know you may be a fall risk. Some hospitals have patients who have trouble getting around wear yellow socks when in the hospital (ask if your hospital's color system is different). This way, anyone who enters the room knows they need assistance walking.

Fall-proof your space

To prevent falls during your hospital stay, keep an eye out for potential hazards like wires, IV poles, loose blankets, your gown, and nearby tables. These items can create trip hazards in a busy hospital room. If you know that walking is challenging or you're prone to falls, be sure to tell your nurse or another member of your care team right away.

Make sure you get rid of these hazards in your home too. Ask your care team about ways to make your home safer. This can include removing loose rugs, adding non-slip mats, and replacing furniture with wheels, or adding grab bars in key areas, like the shower. You should also have someone declutter any pathways, which can lead to trips and falls.

Fall-proof yourself

Ask your care team if it's worth using a cane, walker, rollator, or other assistive device for added stability and help you find the option that works best for you. Gear up right and use non-slip socks and or consider shoes without laces and straps or snaps to avoid tripping.

If you've been falling more often, physical therapy might help build your balance and strength.

TIP

Continue to assess the "fall-proofing" modifications you have and if you need more (or less) support as time goes on. Let your care team more if you are falling more often and where this is happening. Keep the conversation open.

Learn to fall safely

Yes, this is a thing! Professionals like physical therapists can teach you how to fall in a way that minimizes injury risk. They'll teach you how to brace yourself or land safely to reduce the probability of broken bones and concussions. They can also help you prevent falls with techniques called balance training.

Keep your care team informed

If you're falling frequently, let your provider know. Even if you don't feel hurt right away, a fall can cause hidden issues that may need checking. Loop in your support system by sharing with a trusted friend or family member if you've had a recent fall. They can help spot hazards and support any preventive measures you put in place.

TIP

Don't assume that more frequent falls means you'll be forced into a nursing home with no questions asked.

Consider using fall detection technology

Look into wearable fall-monitoring tech or alert systems like the Life Alert or ADT medical alert systems. Some automatically notify loved ones or emergency services when you take a tumble. Others have a button that you press if you're experiencing a medical emergency (see Figure 14-2). Many of these systems are covered by Medicare, so do your research.

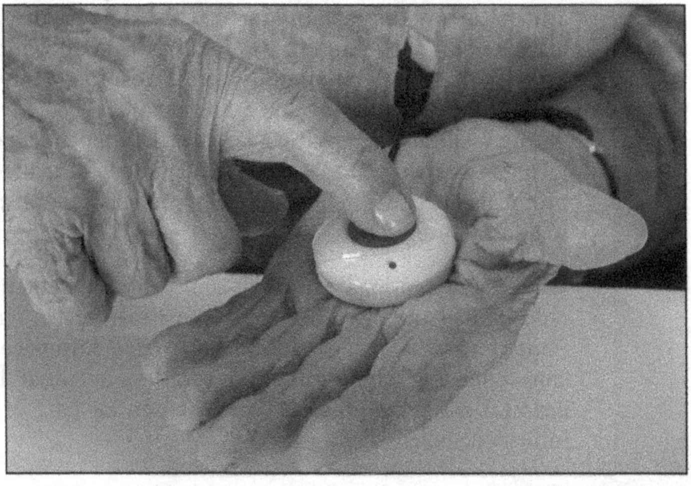

AndreyPopov/Getty Images

FIGURE 14-2: Medical alert bracelets can be a huge help, especially if you live alone.

At the hospital, you may be designated a "fall risk" for the duration of your visit, which usually includes wearing a specific wristband. This designation ensures that extra support is available to help you move safely throughout the hospital. Remember, the more your healthcare team knows about your needs, the better they can assist in keeping you safe.

Understanding Hospital Safety Ratings

Did you know hospitals receive "grades" based on their safety and care quality? It's true! Hospital safety ratings evaluate aspects like infection control, patient falls, and other critical measures. They give patients and consumers insight into the care standards at different facilities.

A parallel to be drawn here could car safety ratings from the National Highway Traffic Safety Administration (NHTSA). In the same way car safety scores reflect how well a car protects passengers in a crash, hospital ratings help give you an idea as to how safe a hospital is.

Hospitals undergo evaluations on things like infection rates, patient satisfaction scores, and mortality rates associated with particular medical procedures. These ratings don't just influence a hospital's public reputation; they can impact insurance reimbursements, accreditation, the ability to attract top healthcare talent, and overall community trust. Hospital safety ratings are useful tools for choosing where to get care, especially when comparing facilities for specific needs or treatments. Looking at these ratings can help you assess how well a hospital adheres to safety protocols, its staff-to-patient ratios, and its general commitment to quality care.

While safety ratings offer valuable insights, remember they're only part of the picture — personal experiences, recommendations, and other considerations may also influence your decision. Choosing where to receive care is a personal decision, but hospital safety ratings can be an essential part of making an informed choice.

FIND ONLINE

Check resources like *U.S. News & World Report* (`https://health.usnews.com/best-hospitals`), Leapfrog's Hospital Safety Guide (`https://www.hospitalsafetygrade.org/`), or CMS Hospital Compare (`www.cms.gov/medicare/quality/initiatives/hospital-quality-initiative/hospital-compare`) to see hospital ratings. You can filter by location, specialty, and other relevant factors. To make the most of these ratings, compare multiple facilities and look for specific metrics that matter to you, such as specialty care or surgical safety.

Advocating for Your Personal Safety

One of the most crucial aspects of patient self-advocacy is accepting that, ultimately, no one but you is fully responsible for ensuring your safety. People can't read minds, and as overwhelmed as the healthcare system is, healthcare professionals are not going to try to read yours.

While healthcare professionals and support systems are dedicated to providing quality care within their roles, it's up to you to make sure you are safe, heard, and fully informed throughout every step of your care.

The same mindset applies to protecting your personal safety in the healthcare system. Keep these fundamental point in mind:

» **Know your rights:** Without knowing your rights including informed consent you cannot identify threats to them nor learn how to protect them.

» **Be familiar with the resources that are there to keep you safe:** Patient advocates, ombudsman offices, and reputable online resources like the CDC, WHO, and `Medicare.gov` can support you in navigating everything from simple questions to complex healthcare decisions.

» **Communicate with your care team:** I wish I could write this in all capital letters, but I don't want to scream at you. Get comfortable expressing your concerns, asking questions, and making requests to your healthcare providers. Clear communication, coupled with your knowledge of your rights and resources, will help you control your healthcare outcomes and empower you.

» **Take personal responsibility for your safety:** Even for processes shared with your healthcare team, be proactive. Ask providers to sanitize their hands before they examine you, confirm your information before a medication is administered to you, and be assertive about identifying and resolving any safety issues that arise. You are your first line of defense.

By understanding your rights, accessing resources, communicating clearly, and taking an active role in your own care, you'll be well-prepared to navigate the healthcare system safely and effectively.

5

Tackling Specialized Patient Advocacy

IN THIS PART . . .

Championing your child's health as a parent advocate

Planning for holistic and compassionate care for aging loved ones

Honing your role as a mental health advocate and getting the support you need

Working with providers to manage end-of-life care

IN THIS CHAPTER

» Understanding the uniqueness of the parent advocate role

» Managing your child's healthcare as they grow

» Communicating your child's needs in educational settings

» Teaching your child to advocate for themselves

» Prioritizing self-care and wellness to combat advocacy fatigue and burnout

Chapter 15
Learning to Champion Your Child's Health

Navigating the healthcare system with your child can feel overwhelming, especially when you're not a healthcare professional. Even if you know how the healthcare system works, chances are you'll sometimes feel like you were dropped into a maze without a map. You are your child's strongest advocate — and your role is crucial to ensuring they receive the best care possible.

This chapter explains what it means to be a parent advocate, and how you can assume the role with confidence. You'll learn strategies for working with professionals involved in your child's care. This chapter also discusses how to empower your child to speak up in conversations about their health so they can play an active role in their healthcare journey.

Advocating for your child's health is a big responsibility — yet it's probably something you already manage in various other parts of their life. This chapter helps you navigate the world of pediatric patient advocacy so you can improve your child's experience with the healthcare system.

Handling Pediatric Advocacy as Children Grow

The care and advocacy needs of children are very different from those of adults. Children think, communicate, and respond to treatment differently. Pediatric medicine, in fact, is a specialized field dedicated to addressing these unique needs.

In pediatric care, providers recognize that children are not just "small adults" — they have their own nuanced medical needs. Their bodies process medications differently, and developmental milestones, like puberty, affect their conditions and responses to treatments that differs from clinical care for adults. Even symptoms may look completely different in children compared to adults, which means providers must consider many unique factors to ensure safe and effective care for kids.

Patient advocacy for children looks different than for adults. Pediatric advocacy often involves multiple layers of communication. As a parent, you'll find that your advocacy style will change as your child grows. You'll need to adjust your approach to best fit the needs and development of your child. Kids change a lot throughout their childhood and adolescence, so the way they communicate and interact with the world.

REMEMBER

Every child is different, and the frequency of these changes in advocacy may vary widely depending on their unique development. For children and individuals with developmental disabilities, these changes can look different, with a pace and type of advocacy that aligns with their own developmental needs.

Each stage of childhood development — from infancy to adolescence — brings unique healthcare needs and ways of interacting with the system. A child's individual genetic makeup, developmental milestones, and growing independence mean their healthcare must adapt more frequently. Whether you're focused on preventive care and wellness visits or navigating a chronic condition, recognizing and responding to your child's distinct needs at each stage is key to supporting their journey.

Accommodating developmental sensitivity

As your child grows and move through stages like infancy, toddlerhood, adolescence, and the teenage years, the way they interact with their healthcare team — and the kind of advocacy they need from you — will naturally shift. It's essential to set realistic expectations for you and your child about treatment plans as they evolve.

A mindset that's sensitive to your child's developmental stages supports safer, more effective interventions that respect a child's changing needs, helping you and your child's providers work together to prioritize the child's long-term health and well-being.

TIP

Ask your child's healthcare team about how current and future treatment plans are expected to change over time. While no one can predict exactly how treatment will shift as your child ages, starting these conversations early can give you a helpful outline of what to anticipate.

Here are some key benefits to discussing this process early:

- **You gain clarity on how your child might respond to treatment as they grow.** As children age, their bodies may respond differently to medications and treatments — especially those intended for long-term use. Talk with your child's provider about how treatment plans might need adjustment as your child develops. For example, some dosages may need to be weight-dependent, or treatment might need to change if it becomes less effective over time. Factors like organ maturity, hormone levels, and body weight could impact treatment effectiveness, so having these discussions early helps you and your provider keep an eye on any signs or symptoms that could signal the need for adjustments in the future.
- **You are prioritizing identification of treatment risks relative to physical development.** By recognizing the dynamic nature of your child's growth and development, you can actively work with their healthcare team to understand both the current treatment plan and how it may evolve as your child reaches new milestones. Understanding the potential risks of treatment as your child develops physically and psychologically is essential.

» **You can comfortably have informed conversations about developmentally appropriate pain management.** Pain management can be a big part of your child's care plan, and it may need to change as your child grows. Children feel and show pain in different ways as they age. For example, infants might only be able to cry when they're in pain, but an older child might be able to tell you where it hurts and describe what it feels like. Talk with your child's healthcare team about how pain management might need to adjust over time. This helps make sure your child's pain is handled in a way that's right for their age and needs, keeping them as comfortable as possible.

TIP

Pain management doesn't always mean using medication. Ask your child's care team ways to manage pain without medication, where appropriate. They can help you find the best techniques for your child and guide you on how to use these methods effectively as part of their care.

» **You are encouraging collaboration with your child's healthcare team.** By actively engaging in conversations with your child's multidisciplinary care team, you're fostering open communication to ensure your child's unique needs are always at the forefront. Discussing how your child's conditions and treatments might evolve over time allows you to frequently stay proactive, rather than reactive, and ensures that your child's personality, preferences, and specific needs are prioritized in their care plan.

These conversations present a chance to start conversations on next steps and strategies if certain changes occur. This level of engagement allows your child's healthcare providers to create a care plan with you and your child that supports their changing clinical needs

Including your child in the informed consent process

Just as in adult care, informed consent is required to authorize any treatment or procedure for your child, ensuring that you understand the purpose, risks, alternatives, and expected outcomes (see Chapter 4 for more on informed consent). For children, a parent or legal guardian typically gives this consent, as they are legally responsible for them. Another process, often used in pediatric clinical research, is "informed assent" where treatments and other parts of the research protocol are explained in a way the child can understand, gaining their agreement when possible. Informed assent is not legally binding, but it is used to make sure that the child is included conversation and interventions about their health.

Here are some key benefits of including your child in the informed consent process:

» **Your child understands what a procedure or test entails.** In an age-appropriate way, your child has the opportunity to understand why they are completing the procedure and what to expect. This minimizes surprise and the fear of the unknown. Empowering children by acknowledging their perspectives builds confidence and sets the groundwork for self-advocacy as they mature.

» **Your child can express their concerns and ask questions.** Adults have tons of questions about their healthcare — so imagine how many a child must have. Encouraging them to ask questions, voice fears, and seek clarification when they don't understand something helps normalize their involvement in their healthcare.

» **Your child becomes an active participant in their own health.** Including your child in the informed consent process enables them to be an active participant in their health journey. Children are more likely to feel empowered (and in some cases, may be more cooperative) when they have some understanding of what's happening to them.

TIP

Invite your child to ask if they're unsure about anything and ask their care team to use simple language and concepts. Pediatric providers and child life specialists are adept at breaking down complex information into digestible bits for children; if clarity is needed, don't hesitate to ask for more.

Supporting your child's emotional and psychological needs

Whether your child is simply attending wellness visits or navigating a serious or chronic illness, consider how mental and emotional health impacts their overall well-being and resilience. Just like adults, children can feel scared, confused, or overwhelmed in the healthcare system. Ensuring they have access to mental health resources that are age-appropriate and suitable for their development and condition can make a big difference in how they cope with and understand their medical experiences.

Navigating healthcare can be challenging — even adults can feel lost trying to communicate their needs to healthcare professionals who use unfamiliar terms and juggle numerous priorities. While children may not fully understand the importance of self-advocacy, they can still experience troubling emotions about where they fit into their care. Talking to your child's healthcare team about when to introduce mental health support can help build emotional resilience early on. See Figure 15-1.

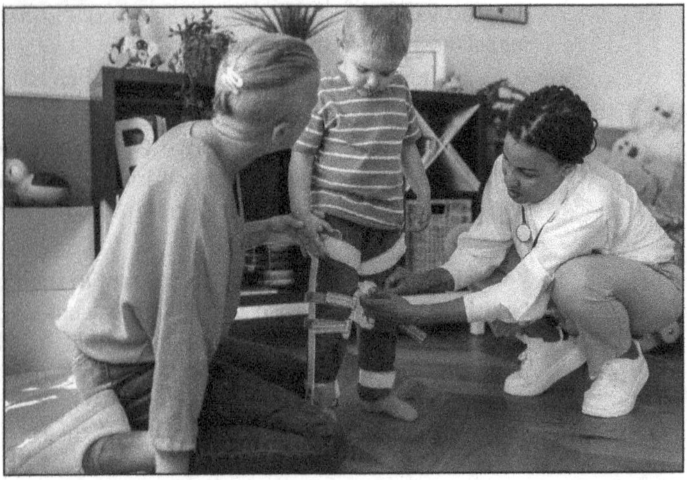

Pekic/Getty Images

FIGURE 15-1: Helping your child become comfortable with their caregivers and their interventions is a good start.

As children grow, they'll face common challenges like peer pressure, stress, and even bullying — all of which can affect their mental health and how they approach their healthcare experiences. Partnering with mental health professionals from an early age can equip your child with tools to manage these challenges, process emotions, and feel more confident and secure inside and outside of a healthcare setting. This support not only aids in handling their current experiences but also prepares them to navigate life's complexities with greater resilience and understanding.

- **Why it matters:** Just like plants need sunlight and water, kids need mental and emotional support to grow strong and healthy. It's not just about fixing problems — it's about helping kids handle their feelings and navigate challenges.
- **When to start:** Don't wait for a crisis. It's like brushing teeth — you don't wait for a cavity to start brushing, right? Start having conversations early with your child's care team about introducing age-appropriate, supportive voices in your child's life to boost their emotional health.
- **Who can help:** Mental health professionals, such as child psychologists, licensed therapists, and counselors, are like coaches. They guide kids in understanding and managing emotions. Their help can lead to your child feel more confident and secure about having conversations about their health and wellness as they mature.
- **What they might face:** Kids don't only deal with illness; they must tackle big stuff like stress, peer pressure, and bullying, just to name a few. Preparing them early to utilize mental health professionals and resources is like giving them a toolkit to handle these challenges and help you and their clinical care team proactively address issues that could affect their well-being.

TIP

Challenging or uncomfortable experiences in the healthcare system can greatly affect your child's comfort and willingness to engage in future medical care. Talk with your child's care team about recognizing signs of medical anxiety or trauma, and work together to prevent or address these feelings.

Managing Care Through Adolescence and the Transition to Adulthood

As your child grows older, they begin to explore their individuality, speak up for themselves, and make decisions. They start reaching important milestones, like getting a driver's license, landing a job, and gaining more independence. Similar growth can happen in their healthcare journey. In their young adulthood, your child will be able to make decisions for themselves. Building the skills of self-advocacy early on can make this transition smoother.

Teaching self-advocacy skills

You might remember the experience yourself — becoming a young adult and suddenly being responsible for making your own doctor's appointments, managing consent forms, understanding insurance, and leading conversations about your health. Amidst all that independence, you may have longed for the days when your parents or guardians manage those processes for you (or you might have even brought your folks along to the next appointment, just in case).

As a young adult, it's exciting to be seen as a decision-maker after years of following your parent or guardian's lead, but it can also feel overwhelming, especially if you've never had the chance to be involved in these conversations before. Many young adults feel unprepared to navigate the healthcare system independently because they haven't had opportunities to practice communicating their needs or understanding what to expect from their care. See Figure 15-2.

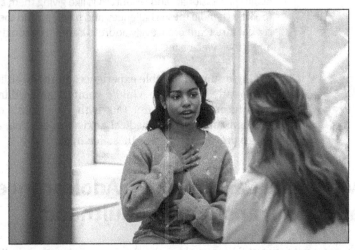

SDI Productions/Getty Images

FIGURE 15-2: Teaching your child to advocate for themselves will reap benefits their whole lives.

The good news? You don't have to wait until your child is 18 to start getting them ready. You can start early, gradually involving them in discussions about their health, encouraging questions, and teaching them how to advocate for themselves.

Consider the following simple steps to help ease them into the driver's seat of their healthcare.

Get them involved early

Start small by letting them ask questions at doctor's appointments or explain how they're feeling. It's a great way to help them feel comfortable speaking up.

Teach the basics

Getting comfortable with the healthcare process takes practice, and starting with small steps can make a big difference. For example, show your child how to call and schedule an appointment. Even if you handle the scheduling, try putting the call on speakerphone or let them dial the number. This way, they get a feel for the process and hear what's involved.

Help them prepare for appointments, too. It's common for people to forget what they wanted to say once they're face-to-face with their provider. Encourage your child to jot down their symptoms, feelings, or questions in a notebook before the appointment. At the visit, let them speak up about their experience, and you can fill in details if needed. This builds their confidence and helps them avoid sitting silently while you recount all their experiences.

As you go through the steps of the "patient day," explain each part. Let them know why you're paying a copay, or what the pharmacist does and encourage them to ask questions. A gradual approach works best. Adopt the mindset of, "I'm showing you this so you'll be able to handle it yourself one day." This can take fear out of the process and give them a sense of independence in managing their own health. Even if they don't grasp everything immediately, familiarity can gradually ease any fear, giving them a solid foundation for the future.

Encourage them to speak up

Emphasize to your child that their feelings and concerns truly matter, and encourage them to practice self-advocacy now, as it will only empower them to do it on their own in the future. After a clinician provides an explanation, take a moment to check if your child understands what they heard. Encourage them to kindly request the clinician or care team to repeat any parts they find unclear, explain what a medication is for, or clarify anything that seems puzzling.

Remind them that seeking answers is important, even if it's merely out of curiosity. Asking questions not only makes them feel more at ease with being involved in their care but also reassures them that it's perfectly acceptable to inquire about their well-being.

TIP

Constructively address behavior, like speaking over the person speaking or name-calling, as it comes up. Help them express big emotions, like fear or anger, with the professionals on their team in helpful ways and reinforce that advocating for yourself doesn't mean being rude or hurtful to the person you're working with, when necessary.

Supporting your child's privacy and confidentiality as they age

Certain aspects of your child's healthcare — like mental health or sexual health — may become private, even before they become a legal adult. Talk with your child's care team about how you can support these aspects of their healthcare while respecting their privacy. This is a way to honor your child as they mature, allowing them to feel safe in trusting and involving you in their care when they choose as they become an adult.

If you're unsure about the rights you and your child have, ask the healthcare team for guidance. Privacy laws, especially for minors, may vary by state, so understanding these nuances can be helpful. You may feel like you are losing visibility into some parts of your child's healthcare, but remember that this is part of their growing independence — and in some cases, it's their legal right. Embracing this shift can support a healthier, more trusting relationship between you and your child as they step into adulthood.

Transitioning from pediatric to adult healthcare providers

At a certain point, your child's care will shift from a pediatric care team to adult healthcare providers. This can be a big change, especially if you and your child have been with the same pediatric providers for years. Your child's pediatrician has probably seen you through their first check-ups and broken bones to everything in between, so this transition can feel like closing a chapter.

With some planning, however, the handoff can be smooth, and your child can build a relationship with an adult healthcare team that's a great fit. It is an opportunity for your child to begin forging a new and supportive relationships with the healthcare providers who will accompany them into adulthood.

Here are a few tips to help ease this transition:

» **Get a head start:** Begin the conversation before your child turns 18 or 21. Talk with the care team about which providers will best support your child's care into adulthood. If your child has a chronic condition and has been seeing a specialist, ask about adult specialists who can continue that care.

» **Get provider recommendations:** Pediatric care teams transition their young adult patients to adult providers all the time. Ask your current pediatric team to suggest adult providers who align well with your child's needs. Ask about their communication style. From here, you can research recommended providers to help assess whether they'll be a good fit.

» **Clarify what changes:** Some pediatric providers may follow patients into young adulthood for certain conditions and disabilities, while other care needs may transition to new providers. Confirm which parts of care will stay with the pediatric team and which will move to adult providers.

» **Interview new providers:** Set up initial appointments with potential adult providers to get a sense of how they communicate and whether you and your child feel comfortable as a trial run. Ask about their experience with similar conditions, and make sure they're open to the communication style that works for you and your child.

» **Gather medical records:** Ensure your child's medical records and other relevant information are shared with the new provider well in advance. This helps create a seamless transition, so the new provider has a complete picture before the first appointment

TIP

Even if you're transitioning to another provider within the same health system or hospital, take time to double-check that all records are accurate and up-to-date. This is a great opportunity to work with your child's providers to make sure that things like old medications or ruled-out conditions are marked as such. This helps make the new provider's review of the chart more straightforward and focused.

» **Establish a strong start:** At the first appointment, share a quick overview of your child's pediatric care journey, what you hope to accomplish with the new provider, and any specific preferences for communication. Discuss scheduling needs, and ask how often you should meet so you can plan appointments in advance.

TIP

If you and your child have specific cultural beliefs that may influence their care or provide important perspectives and context for their healthcare as they transition into adulthood, seek out and prioritize healthcare providers who display cultural sensitivity and understanding. Choosing culturally aware providers can empower your child to confidently navigate their healthcare experiences, because they know that their cultural background is acknowledged and honored throughout their evolving healthcare relationship.

Communicating Your Child's Needs in Educational Settings

For many children, school is one of the most significant environments for social interaction and development. As you navigate your child's healthcare, consider that their medical needs can impact not only their relationship with their clinical care team but also their experience at school.

While the healthcare team provides guidance on treatment, prevention, and recovery, school staff — such as teachers and administrators — play a crucial role in supporting your child's learning experience and adapting as needed to any health challenges.

For most children, school is where they spend a large part of their day, so it's essential to coordinate between your child's healthcare team and their school to ensure they're supported in both spaces.

Here's how you can begin to cultivate this collaboration to ensure a holistic support system:

» **Identify the intersections:** Some medical needs may impact how your child participates in school, requiring accommodations to support their learning and social development. Start conversations with both your child's healthcare providers and school staff to discuss what accommodations could look like. For example, a child with attention deficit hyperactivity disorder (ADHD) might benefit from taking tests in quieter environments or having extra time for assignments.

- **Learn the process for getting accommodations:** Get familiar with the steps to set up and manage accommodations or education plans such as an Individualized Education Plan (IEP) or 504 Plan, if needed. Ask your child's school for guidance on the accommodations they recommend and how to mobilize a plan to address them. Ask what documentation or doctor's notes need to be presented, how frequently they need to be renewed, and what the administrative process for modifying them would be.
- **Create a feedback loop:** Establish regular communication between your child's healthcare providers, educators, and yourself. For example, if your child's teachers notice they're struggling to focus, seem unengaged, or not managing pain well, keep an open line of communication so you can share this information with your child's healthcare providers as well and adjust the support plan as needed.
- **Utilize school resources:** In addition to teachers, explore other school resources. The school nurse, for instance, can help make sure medication schedules are adhered to during school hours, and special education professionals can work with your child's care team to tailor support.
- **Anticipate change:** As your child's healthcare needs evolve, keep both healthcare and education teams informed. For instance, if a surgical procedure is planned, discuss post-surgery educational support with the healthcare team to determine appropriate adaptations needed from the school. They can also offer advice on the kinds of adjustments to request from the school.
- **Set goals and track observations:** Take note of any observations you make at home, such as if your child struggles with homework or seems to zone out. Write down these observations and bring them up with both the healthcare and education teams. Even small details can be important to understanding your child's needs and tailoring their support to meet goals for their care in the future.

REMEMBER

Each child's needs are unique, and these conversations are likely to evolve over time. Don't hesitate to reach out to your child's healthcare team for advice on how to communicate with the school. Pediatric providers are often experienced in helping families work with educators because they understand that school is a significant part of a child's life.

TIP

If you're concerned about developmental milestones, or if something doesn't seem quite right, trust your instincts and ask questions. Pediatric teams understand that children change at different rates and aim to support your child's well-being and success across all facets of life.

Teaching Your Child to Advocate for Their Health

Teaching your child how to advocate for their health is as essential as teaching them stranger danger or saying "please" and "thank you." One day, they'll need to have challenging conversations about their health on their own. Here are some tips to get them started on this journey with confidence:

- **Introduce self-advocacy early:** Explain patient advocacy in simple terms — encourage your child to speak up when they don't understand something and remind them that doctors and nurses are part of their team. Ask their providers to reinforce that their voice matters. When authority figures encourage questions, it helps kids feel that their input is as valuable as their providers'.
- **Have them practice speaking up:** Encourage open communication of needs. For example, if your child is feeling cold, suggest they ask for a blanket. If they struggle with swallowing pills, encourage them to inform the clinician and explore alternatives. These interactions foster confidence, making your child an active participant in their healthcare.
- **Teach them to express feelings openly:** If they're experiencing discomfort, encourage them to say, "My arm hurts when I move it this way," or "I need a break." Reinforce their openness with responses by acknowledging their communication by saying thing like, "Thank you for telling me," or

"Sure, we can take a break" and ask providers to do the same. This helps normalize expressing needs and asking for support.

- **Foster curiosity:** Motivate your child to be inquisitive about their health and to ask questions. Reassure them that curiosity is welcomed, and collaborate with the care team to provide explanations in relatable terms. Encourage follow-up questions to aid their understanding of information.
- **Model curiosity:** Show them that you, too, ask questions about their care. Demonstrating curiosity helps them understand that it's okay — and important — to ask questions about health matters. Showing your own curiosity underscores the importance and normalcy of asking questions about health, and it cultivates a learning environment.
- **Acknowledge assertiveness:** Celebrate moments when your child respectfully communicates, whether by saying, "Excuse me, I have a question," or waiting their turn to speak. Your encouragement builds a comfortable atmosphere for future healthcare interactions.
- **Educate them on roles in healthcare:** When they encounter new healthcare team members, encourage your child to inquire about each person's role. This helps demystify the system and might even spark an interest in healthcare professions.
- **Encourage them to stay in tune with their body:** Help your child notice and describe their symptoms. If they have a headache, prompt them to describe how it feels. Noticing these cues teaches them to understand their body's signals and communicate them clearly to get the right support.
- **Let them make age-appropriate decisions:** Encourage your child to make small choices about their care, like picking the color of their cast or choosing a medication flavor. Gradually introduce decision-making to help them weigh options and consider future outcomes.
- **Engage them in simple learning moments:** Encourage them to ask the clinician to explain things like an x-ray or other basic visuals. Let them see an x-ray of their broken arm before and after their cast goes on to help normalize the conversation around their care.

» **Adapt based on your child's needs:** Use your judgment to tailor these strategies, ensuring your child's comfort and safety. Your guidance today will help them grow into an active participant in their healthcare, building skills that may serve them (and even you!) sooner than expected.

Encouraging your child to actively participate in their healthcare experience while they are young gives them a head-start at being a successful, self-advocating patient in the future.

TIP

Make health literacy a priority. Ask your providers to explain complex topics in clear, everyday language, and seek out resources that build your child's understanding of health basics. Consider age-appropriate books, educational TV shows, or YouTube series to help lay a solid foundation they grow.

Staying Well on the Pediatric Advocacy Journey

The process of standing by your child's side as they navigate the healthcare system and work with healthcare providers is truly a journey. Throughout the course of your supporting your child, you will watch your child go through very difficult and scary moments where they will be relying on you and on the relationships you've fostered with their healthcare providers to keep them safe, and hopefully make them well. Many parents and guardians have responsibilities to other people and children as well. Needless to say, this awesome responsibility can be stressful.

Although it might seem impractical to chalk out time in your day for yourself so that you can be the best parent, guardian, or advocate for your child, it can also be important. At the end of the day, your child gets one you. Even if there are other loving people in their support network who help and support them, they need you. If you don't get the rest and downtime you need, you can't act in their best interest.

This section reviews the importance of having a support network for you and your child and provides you with some tips and tricks for considering your own wellness along the way.

Recognizing advocacy fatigue and burnout

While your role as an advocate is crucial, the emotional and physical demands of advocating for your child can sometimes feel like scaling a mountain without rest. Remaining constantly attentive about managing your child's healthcare can lead to what's known as *advocacy fatigue*. This state of feeling drained, frazzled, or emotionally depleted from tirelessly striving to secure the best possible care for your child. This feeling is not uncommon and certainly doesn't tarnish your standing as a caring parent or guardian — it just makes you human.

Here are some telltale signs and soothing strategies to manage advocacy fatigue:

- **Trouble concentrating during appointments:** If you're zoning out or struggling to keep up in conversations with your child's healthcare team, it might be more than just missing your morning coffee. Feeling exhausted and unfocused can be a sign that you're burning out.
- **Avoiding in-depth discussions:** Do you dread discussing upcoming appointments or treatment plans? These conversations can take a lot out of you, mentally and emotionally. Advocacy fatigue can make even routine planning feel overwhelming, leading you to avoid these important conversations.
- **Noticing new physical problems:** Noticeable headaches, changes in digestive health, or constant tiredness might be your body's way of waving a red flag — a physical response to the stress tied to having to be "on" all the time. Meet with your own doctor to investigate further.
- **Relying too much on healthcare providers' decisions:** At times, you might find yourself overly deferring to the healthcare team's decisions because the weight of contributing is just too much. This could be a sign to pause and recharge.
- **Experiencing emotional shifts:** Increased frustration or anxiety from the continuous responsibility of advocating for your child could be a sign of fatigue that shouldn't be ignored.

REMEMBER

It's completely understandable to feel fatigued when advocating for your child's health. You're not a bad person — you're just human. Taking care of yourself is a way of taking care of your child. Fill up the cup you pour from.

Combating advocacy fatigue

Taking care of your child's health is incredibly rewarding, yet it can also be quite overwhelming at times. Here are some practical tips to navigate advocacy fatigue and maintain your own wellness while supporting your child's healthcare journey:

- **Create a daily game plan:** Rather than feeling burdened by an endless to-do list, try breaking down responsibilities into daily, manageable tasks. For instance, dedicate Monday to refilling prescriptions and scheduling future appointments. On Tuesday, assist your child in getting ready for their Wednesday visit. Tackling smaller tasks each day can help you feel more in control of your day and ensure a steady progress.
- **Ask for guidance when you need it:** If you find larger tasks daunting, don't hesitate to seek advice from your child's healthcare team on where to begin. You might also consider hiring a professional private patient advocate to help plan and organize your tasks effectively.
- **Set time aside for yourself:** As hard as it sounds, schedule dedicated time for yourself each day or week to do something that supports your wellness. Whether it's going for a jog, practicing meditation, reading, catching up on a favorite show, or meeting friends for coffee, giving yourself this mental break, time for yourself can renew your energy and resilience, allowing you to be more present for your child.
- **Practice self-compassion:** Remember, no one expects perfection. The fact that you're taking steps to improve your child's healthcare experience shows how much you care. When self-criticism creeps in, try to stop the negative spiral and remind yourself of the dedication you're bringing to a challenging role.
- **Find an accountability partner and build a support network:** If self-criticism or doubt becomes overwhelming, consider asking a friend or family member to serve as an accountability partner. They can help you regain focus and

remind you of the tremendous job you're doing. Having someone supportive can make a substantial difference. In many cases, being an advocate to your child is just one of the many name tags you wear and have other responsibilities in life as well. Communicate with your friends and family and lean on them if you need help with things like meal prepping or cooking, picking something up from the store, or other small errands. The people that care about your child probably care about you too and would be more than happy to pitch in where necessary to help reduce your stress so that you can focus on what your child needs. Consider connecting with other parents or guardians that are walking a similar path as you and your child to have a sense of community, learn something, and even provide and be provided encouragement.

TIP

Consider investing in professional mental health support as well. If you're comfortable, ask your child's pediatric care team if they have parent support programs and professionals to connect you with as you support your child. Millions of parents and guardians are in the same boat, so you might even be able to find community.

- **Give yourself grace for your mistakes:** It's perfectly natural to feel uncertain or make mistakes along the way. Forgetting to cancel an appointment or feeling confused about the next course of action doesn't make you a "bad" parent — it makes you human. Acknowledge that mistakes happen and give yourself the grace to keep moving forward. No one expects perfection.

IN THIS CHAPTER

» Planning for holistic care in senior needs

» Getting the legal paperwork in order

» Respecting an aging loved one's humanity

Chapter 16
Managing Compassionate Care for Aging Loved Ones

If you've ever had the privilege of having a conversation with an elder, you've likely heard them say that growing older is an experience all its own. Each person's journey through aging is unique, shaped by the life they've led, the perspectives they've cultivated, and the changes they've experienced. While you may not consider yourself advanced in age, think back to your teenage years — what's changed mentally, physically, and emotionally since then? You can probably make a list of how you've changed with age. Priorities shift with time; things that didn't matter as much in your youth often take on new significance.

The support patients need as they age varies widely, influenced by factors like lifelong health, current physical and mental condition, and individual preferences. For an aging loved one, navigating healthcare involves more than just physical changes — it encompasses years of experiences, the tapestry of their lives, and lessons that have shaped their perspective.

This chapter explores the value of holistic care planning tailored to the specific needs of seniors. It discusses the importance of respecting their choices and treating them as a person, not just as a patient, and includes ways to legally safeguard their care preferences. You learn strategies to understand their goals and priorities, ensuring that as they age, their dignity and desires remain at the forefront of their healthcare journey.

Preparing a Holistic Plan for Senior Care Needs

When it comes to senior care, the "one-size-fits-all" approach just doesn't cut it. Effective care should reflect a person's unique needs, goals, and expectations, with the flexibility to evolve as circumstances change.

Personalizing care ensures comprehensive well-being, covering aspects like physical health, emotional support, social connections, and mental health. Even if certain needs remain consistent, a patient's priorities can shift, so flexibility is key.

To build a customized care plan, start by working with your loved one and their healthcare team to understand their full spectrum of needs — clinical, emotional, social, and beyond. Involve your loved one as much as possible in these decisions. For adult children and guardians, remember that part of your role is to respect and uphold their wishes to the best of your ability.

TIP

Having a current, organized list of their providers, along with each provider's goals and objectives, can make care coordination smoother, even when the team keeps expanding.

Patient care requires a team approach. Aim to keep all providers aligned to the care goals, and if you're feeling overwhelmed, don't hesitate to identify areas where you need additional support. Ask yourself:

- Is time to dedicate to the coordination of care an issue?
- Are certain providers difficult to connect with?
- Are certain team members communicating less effectively than others?

By addressing these challenges head-on, you can more easily locate resources, such as adult day programs, to support your loved one's needs.

Aging does not automatically equate to illness; many seniors lead independent lives, while others may need more support. Regular evaluations and updates to the care plan, based on current health and objectives, help maintain its relevance and adaptability. These conversations should be ongoing, involving your loved one and their healthcare team.

A strong relationship with a primary care provider (PCP) becomes even more valuable as your loved one ages. A PCP familiar with your loved one's overall health needs can be a crucial ally.

TIP

Consider adding a geriatrician to your loved one's care team. Geriatricians are trained to understand the unique aspects of senior health, from medication management to age-specific care considerations, and they can be a wonderful resource.

Taking on the Role of a Durable Power of Attorney

A durable healthcare power of attorney is a legal document that designates a person — someone your loved one trusts — to make medical decisions on their behalf if they're unable to do so themselves.

It's important to officially appoint someone in this role because, otherwise, it can be unclear who has legal authority to make decisions for the elderly person. That's true even if you're a constant presence at their appointments, the staff knows you by name, and your loved one's healthcare team has come to recognize you as their go-to person. It may feel like you're already "the one" to step in if needed, but without the right legal documents, that may not be the case. Legally, the authority to make decisions doesn't automatically belong to the person who is most present — it could fall to a spouse, adult child, or even someone else in the family.

Creating a formal healthcare power of attorney ensures that your loved one's wishes are clearly outlined and that a trusted person, not someone assigned by default, will make decisions if they're unable to do so.

In addition to assigning a power of attorney, it's a good idea to discuss these other legal documents:

- **Living wills:** Written, legal documents that outline the person's wishes regarding medical care, or for the termination of medical support in certain circumstances. They indicate their wishes for the use or discontinuation of life-sustaining treatments. They're used if a person becomes incapacitated and is unable to communicate the way they normally do.
- **DNR (Do Not Resuscitate) orders:** These are legally recognized orders signed by a doctor at the patient's request and indicate that the patient does not want to be resuscitated if they suddenly go into cardiac arrest or stop breathing. These are more common for people with a terminal condition or whose chance of surviving resuscitation is low.

In emergencies, these documents can provide crucial guidance. Chapter 18 has more about these important documents.

If you're appointed as a healthcare power of attorney:

- **Take the time to understand your responsibilities thoroughly:** Make sure copies of the power of attorney documentation are on file with your loved one's healthcare providers and are accessible to their care team.
- **Know exactly what your role entails:** Especially in areas like financial and legal matters, as this is key to acting in your loved one's best interest.

If anything is unclear, consider consulting an attorney for guidance on the full scope of your rights and responsibilities in this role.

Advocating for an Aging Loved One Without Minimizing Their Humanity

As your loved one ages or their care needs intensify, you may find yourself taking on a more central role in managing their care. Even with the best of intentions, it can be easy to slip into the habit of speaking for them — or over them — during interactions with their healthcare team.

It's crucial to remember the importance of validating your loved one's position and autonomy in their care. Many older adults have spent much of their lives advocating for others, perhaps even for you, and they likely value being respected and heard in return.

Your intent may be to help, but it's equally essential to ensure that your delivery and approach honor their voice and dignity.

Consider small but impactful ways to ensure their voice is prioritized:

- Avoid speaking over them.
- Give them time to answer questions on their own.
- Allow room for their thoughts and desires to be shared uninterrupted and give them the time they need to share their thoughts.
- Refrain from positioning yourself as the "one who knows best."

Chances are, your loved one already values your judgment and advice; it's about reciprocating that trust.

TIP

Sometimes it's helpful to take a step back and remember who your loved one is as a person, beyond their current healthcare needs. Whether it's your mom, dad, or grandparent, trust in their ability to know themselves and what they want from their care. If your loved one has cognitive impairments or other factors that affect their ability to make their own decision, work with their care team to identify the best action.

REMEMBER

Advocacy means supporting someone's best interests and wishes — not overshadowing them with your perspective. Even if you don't agree with their choices, let them know you respect their decision and ask how they'd like you to support them in seeing it through.

IN THIS CHAPTER

- » Treating mental health as a medical condition
- » Advocating for yourself when your treatment isn't working
- » Getting the mental health support you need

Chapter 17

Bridging the Gap in Mental Health Advocacy

The stigma around mental health disease often creates barriers for patients who are seeking support, making an already challenging healthcare journey feel even more isolating. For those managing mental health conditions — conditions that are real, valid, and often manageable — the struggle to receive appropriate care can feel like an uphill battle, with the healthcare system and even some providers not fully recognizing their needs.

This chapter includes insights to help you navigate conversations about mental health with your providers. The goal is to empower you to advocate for the care and respect you deserve.

Recognizing Mental Health Conditions as Medical Conditions

Mental health conditions are medical conditions — full stop. They require the same level of care, attention, and medical support as any physical health condition. The goal is also the same — to help patients achieve the best possible outcome and quality of life. If you or a loved one is living with a mental health condition, it's essential to acknowledge the validity of what they are experiencing, the impact on their daily life, and the need for comprehensive care.

Did you know, according to NAMI (`nami.org`), that:

- 1 in 5 U.S. adults experience mental illness each year
- 1 in 20 U.S. adults experience serious mental illness each year
- 1 in 6 U.S. youth aged 6-17 experience a mental health disorder each year
- 50 percent of all lifetime mental illness begins by age 14, and 75 percent begin by age 24

All too often, mental health issues are minimized or dismissed as personal failings rather than respected as genuine medical concerns. This stigma is a major reason that disparities in mental healthcare persist.

Recognizing your experience — whether it involves depression, anxiety, schizophrenia, or another mental health condition — and advocating for proper treatment is a vital first step.

Addressing the stigma is challenging, as it's deeply rooted in societal perceptions and can be further compounded by cultural factors. For example, some communities of color face additional stigma around mental health, with family and friends sometimes regarding these conditions as something that can simply be overcome with willpower or minor lifestyle changes.

REMEMBER

It's worth emphasizing that while lifestyle changes and practices like meditation can certainly complement mental health treatment, they are not always the sole solution. The key is proper diagnosis and professional mental health support. Just as medication is necessary for managing chronic conditions like hypertension, medication may also be essential to handling certain mental health conditions. Both are valid medical needs.

Advocating for yourself can include reshaping your perspective on mental health, educating those around you when appropriate, and standing firm in your right to comprehensive, respectful care. You don't owe anyone an explanation for seeking the care you need!

WARNING

You don't have to take this journey alone. If you're having suicidal thoughts, reach out. The U.S. national suicide and crisis hotline number is 988. You can also reach out to the National Suicide Prevention Lifeline at 1-800-273-TALK (8255) or text CSIS to 839863. In Canada, the hotline number is 1-888-353-2273.

Finding Harmony Between Your Health Goals and Your Safety

When setting mental health goals, think of them like any health goal — challenging but within reach. For instance, a patient with a heart condition might dream of exercising more but knows that it requires gradual steps, under a doctor's guidance, rather than suddenly starting a vigorous exercise regimen. Approaching mental health goals in a similar way ensures your safety and helps build sustainable progress.

Start by sharing your ultimate goal, your "North Star," with your provider. This gives them a clear understanding of where you want to be and allows them to create a plan with realistic, safe steps toward that goal. Just as you'd ask your surgeon if it's safe to put weight on your leg after an operation, ask your mental health professional about the impact of certain actions on your mental health journey. They can guide you on what steps are safe to take now and what might require further progress.

Keep in mind that some goals might be out of reach at the moment, and that's okay. It's valuable to have open conversations with your provider about the timing and steps for achieving those goals when it's appropriate and safe.

Telling Your Clinician that Your Treatment Plan Isn't Working

If a treatment or medication you initially received isn't working as expected or is causing side effects, it's essential to speak up. Advocating for yourself ensures that your care team knows if a treatment plan isn't achieving its intended results or if new issues are surfacing.

Don't feel pressured to "tough it out." Your feedback about how you're tolerating the treatment and how you're feeling is crucial to keeping you safe and supported.

REMEMBER

Even when you have a serious mental health condition, you still have the right to advocate for your own care. However, if you find advocating for yourself challenging or an undue burden and you are clearly in over your head, consider giving a trusted loved one power of attorney to make decisions for you or working with a private patient advocate who specializes in mental health advocacy. Chapter 16 talks more about using the power of attorney effectively in your healthcare journey.

Even if a side effect feels minor, don't hesitate to mention it. For example, if the medication is making you jittery or overly fatigued, communicate this directly. Let your provider know exactly what you're experiencing — describe when it happens, how long it lasts, how it affects your daily life, and ask if there are alternatives. Often, there might be options such as adjusting dosages, trying different medications, or considering alternative therapies. Sometimes it takes multiple medications before you find the one that works best, so don't be afraid to speak up.

If you're working with a therapist and find it challenging to stay engaged, bring this up. Ask if there are ways to make the sessions more meaningful or aligned with your needs. Providers appreciate when patients express what is or isn't working — this feedback helps tailor care.

Advocating for Solutions that Increase Your Quality of Life

Our mental health significantly impacts your quality of life. When symptoms aren't well-managed or increase, they can interfere with daily activities and the things we love to do. Approaching mental health solutions holistically can improve well-being and help people integrate positive practices into their everyday routines.

Work with your providers to find ways to incorporate their guidance into things you already enjoy. For instance, if your provider suggests getting more rest, meditating, or staying hydrated, think of realistic ways to add these into your day. Maybe that's keeping a water bottle on your nightstand to drink first thing in the morning or setting a daily reminder for a five-minute mindfulness break during lunch. If you're unsure about where to begin with holistic practices, ask your provider for simple recommendations.

TIP

Community can be a powerful support. Connecting with others on a similar mental health journey can help you feel seen and understood, which can be especially valuable when you're feeling isolated. Finding community — whether in support groups, online forums, or local gatherings — can make a meaningful difference.

Finding Support from Mental Health Programs

If you're looking for mental health resources and support programs to supplement the work with your care team, a good starting point is to ask your therapist or psychiatrist if there are established groups or programs affiliated with the hospital or care center where you receive treatment.

Beyond your immediate care network, there are also community-based options like peer support groups, hotlines, and online support communities.

FIND ONLINE

The National Alliance on Mental Illness (NAMI) is a respected organization and their website provides lots of good information about mental illness, including warning signs and symptoms, advocacy, and ways to find support and education (see Figure 17-1). Check it out at `www.nami.org`.

You can often find safe, supportive spaces online, including groups on social media where you can connect with others who may be navigating similar experiences. Just remember to approach online communities with caution and ensure they're safe, respectful, and aligned with your needs.

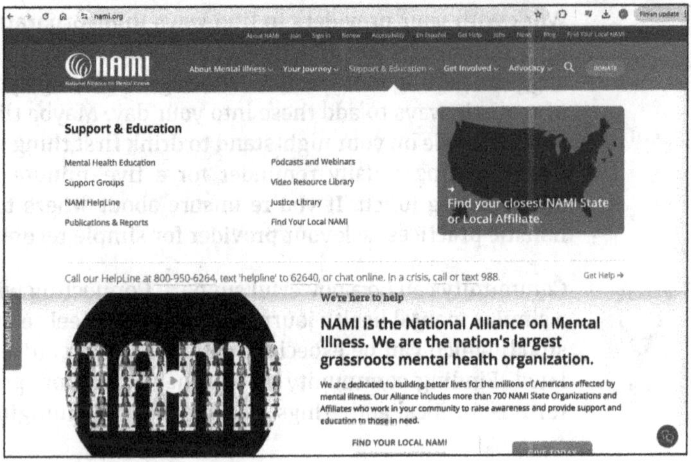

FIGURE 17-1: Check out the National Alliance on Mental Illness (NAMI) website for support.

IN THIS CHAPTER

» Expressing your wishes about end-of-life care

» Getting your legal affairs in order

» Helping your loved one manage end-of-life care with dignity

» Working with providers to manage pain and other symptoms

Chapter 18 Navigating End-of-Life Care

Talking about death and end-of-life planning is rarely easy — it's an inevitable part of life, yet it often feels uncomfortable. However, when these discussions become relevant, whether in your care or when you're caring for a loved one, taking time to clarify what truly matters can be invaluable. This process includes understanding the patient's wishes around end-of-life care, planning for the financial and legal challenges that can arise, and ensuring that these considerations are in place for peace of mind.

This chapter guides you through these meaningful topics, shedding light on essential conversations and choices involved in end-of-life planning.

Understanding and Respecting Wishes at the End of Life

Just as patients have goals and preferences for their other aspects of their healthcare, many also have specific wishes regarding end-of-life care. Discussing these wishes openly with loved ones and healthcare providers is essential for maintaining some control in a process that can feel overwhelmingly unpredictable.

Have a compassionate, honest conversation with your support team about where you'd prefer to be while receiving end-of-life care, what kind of care you envision, and any specific requests you have. If you're the caregiver, you might need to initiate this conversation with your loved one, even if it feels uncomfortable at first to do so. The sooner in their journey you begin these conversations, the better off everyone will be.

Creating an open dialogue also allows family members to ask questions and understand the patient's needs. The goals is to make sure everyone is on the same page when it matters most.

These conversations are understandably difficult, and even for professionals who work in end-of-life care regularly, they recognize the gravity of the moment for each patient. Be sure to communicate your views about medical interventions, like life-sustaining measures and pain management, and take time to think through your options. The most important thing is to avoid leaving these decisions unaddressed, only for loved ones to be left guessing later. Start with what you feel comfortable discussing, knowing that it's okay if your preferences evolve over time. As you clarify your wishes, ensure your care team is informed and that any necessary legal documents are in place to protect those decisions.

If you're open to it, involve family members and close friends in these discussions. Their presence can provide support that you might not have realized you needed, strengthening the sense of unity and understanding as you plan for what lies ahead.

Legal Documents: Power of Attorneys, Living Wills, and More

Talking about your end-of-life care preferences is crucial, but to ensure your wishes are respected, you'll need to put certain legal documents in place. Here are some important terms you may encounter during this process:

- **Advance directive:** This document gives clear instructions to healthcare providers regarding a patient's specific care wishes for their future clinical care, including end-of-life. Documents like DNRs/DNI and healthcare proxies are types of advance directives.
- **DNR (Do Not Resuscitate) orders:** These are legally recognized orders signed by a doctor at the patient's request and they indicate that the patient does not want to be resuscitated if they suddenly go into cardiac arrest or stop breathing. These are more common for people with a terminal condition or whose chance of surviving resuscitation is low.
- **Living will:** This document details which treatments a patient wants to receive or avoid. It can be very helpful for loved ones, because it provides clear guidance on a loved one's preferences when they cannot express them themselves. Preferences on artificial nutrition, organ donation, and spiritual or religious beliefs are outlined here.
- **Healthcare proxy:** Also called a healthcare power of attorney, this is a person the patient designates to make medical decisions on their behalf if they are unable to make them for themselves. This person is usually someone who knows the patient very well.

TIP

It's best to work with an attorney experienced in healthcare or end-of-life planning to create these documents. Once completed, make sure they're filed with your health system to ensure they're accessible. Documents stored in a drawer or a personal file may not be available when they're needed, so having copies on file with your healthcare providers can make all the difference.

Palliative Care versus Hospice Care and the Transition Between Living Arrangements

As you navigate the healthcare journey, especially in end-of-life care, you might consider transitioning to a new living arrangement, such as moving from your home to a skilled nursing facility or another supportive environment.

Chapter 13 covers long-term care, where you can read about what kind of support each option provides.

It's also essential to understand the difference between palliative care and hospice care. While both provide comfort, they serve different purposes:

- **Palliative care:** Focuses on symptom management and relief for individuals with serious illnesses, whether or not they can be cured. Palliative care can be implemented alongside clinical treatment, like chemotherapy, to increase the patient's quality of life It's available at any stage of illness and isn't restricted to end-of-life care.
- **Hospice care:** Specifically supports those at the end of their lives. Hospice is for individuals whose doctor has given them a life expectancy of six months or less and who have decided to focus solely on comfort rather than curative treatments. Patients in hospice care are no longer undergoing treatment for their condition(s). Hospice care is usually fully covered by health insurance.

Knowing these distinctions can help you make more informed decisions about care options and how each type is covered by insurance.

WARNING

Deciding to shift focus to symptom relief, comfort, or stopping treatments altogether can be deeply emotional for the patient and their support system. Work with your care team to find counseling and support groups that can help everyone involved process feelings of grief, anxiety, and any other emotions that may arise. This support can make a challenging time a bit easier for everyone to navigate.

Practical Matters: Financial Affairs

Finances and healthcare are closely linked, even in end-of-life care. Patients should work with financial and legal professionals, such as tax professionals and estate planning attorneys, to safeguard assets and explore steps like assigning guardianship for dependents, managing possessions, and planning for the distribution of their estate. It may seem minor, but starting these conversations early can help reduce complications later on and can allow decisions to be made with the patient's input.

TIP

Keep all important documents, like insurance policies, property deeds, and other estate-related information, in a secure but accessible location. As the time feels right, appoint an executor and discuss wills and asset distribution with family or your support network and make sure everyone understands the arrangements. This will minimize confusion and support a smooth process during an emotional time.

Managing Pain and Symptom Relief

When end-of-life care is part of your or a loved one's journey, pain management may become a key focus. Collaborate closely with the healthcare team to find the most effective ways to manage immediate and long-term pain, as well as breakthrough pain that can arise unexpectedly. Remember, symptom management isn't always just about managing pain; providers can the patient on non-pharmacological treatments that might help ease other symptoms, such as breathing difficulties or fatigue, and improve overall comfort.

TIP

Make pain and symptom management an ongoing conversation. As a person's condition evolves, their needs may change as well. Adjustments to the treatment regimen may be needed to ensure that they remain effective and provide as much comfort as possible.

Helping Your Loved One Manage End-of-Life with Dignity

The chapter has so far covered end-of-life care mostly from the perspective of you as the patient. However, what if you are helping a loved one manage the dying process and make decisions about end-of-life care? How do you have these conversations and ensure that your loved one's wishes are respected while maintaining their dignity?

Here are a couple of tips to remember about these difficult conversations:

- **Start slow:** Going through this process with a loved one can be difficult for both of you. The entire process is full of emotions, so try not to overwhelm yourself or your loved one with rapid fire questions all at once.
- **Consider any remaining wishes or goals:** Talk to your loved on about what's important to them and whether they have anything they'd like to do or accomplish before they die.
- **Find out what's truly important:** Ask open-ended questions to help your loved one articulate what's truly important to them on this final journey. This can help them recognize what has given their life meaning.
- **Work on recognizing and resolving any conflicts:** If you can, help your loved one enter this stage of their life without regrets or unresolved personal conflicts.

6 The Part of Tens

IN THIS PART . . .

Seeking out professional support when your journey becomes confusing

Advocating for a healthier community outside the hospital

Sharing your health journey with others

Celebrating your wins and milestones

IN THIS CHAPTER

- » Considering a second opinion
- » Dealing with medical malpractice
- » Getting help with your healthcare navigation issues
- » Seeking out counseling and services for mental health
- » Working with a private patient advocate

Chapter 19
Ten Ways to Get Professional Support

So you're doing everything you can to advocate for yourself along your healthcare journey. You've taken the time to understand how to communicate with your providers, you got organized about your approach to preparing for your appointments, but you're banging your head against the wall wondering why you are exhausted. Don't worry! Sometimes, depending on the complexity of the care or personal preference, it makes sense to call in the heavyweights, or professionals, for help.

From considering a second opinion to working with a private patient advocate, this chapter gives you a crash course on how to utilize the valuable expertise of those who have dedicated their career and, in many cases, their lives, to addressing healthcare concerns.

Get a Second Opinion

Once you've received a proposed line of treatment from your clinician, don't be afraid to get a second opinion. Especially when the treatment is an expensive or invasive surgery with a host of potential side-effects, it's wise to get a second opinion from another clinician in the same field.

Sometimes the more options you have to consider, the better, when making an important decision. A good clinician will encourage your need to consider all avenues for treatment. Chapter 11 covers the ups and downs of getting second opinions in more detail.

Work with Legal Professionals

Although healthcare professionals try their best to ensure that patients stay safe from injury, infection, and other preventable illnesses while in their care, injury and malpractice still occur. If you feel that your healthcare experience has involved malpractice or other medical harm, consider consulting with a medical malpractice attorney.

Medical malpractice attorneys are experts in guiding patients, and their families, through the process of substantiating claims of medical negligence and harm with evidence and seeking compensation if there is a case. These legal professionals have an expansive knowledge of personal injury law can be invaluable resources when medical harm is a part of the healthcare experience.

TIP

When you are researching appropriate legal counsel, look for attorneys who specialized in either personal injury law or medical malpractice. It's important to make sure that these professionals are in good standing with the bar association and have positive testimonials or reviews.

Take into account compensation models for each practice to make sure you understand what the expected financial obligations are, even for consultations, and ensure that your budget aligns with them. For example, some law firms don't require payment unless you win your case. Take into account the attorney's professional memberships or affiliations and learn about their track record.

TIP

Before attending your first legal consultation, call the office and ask what you need to provide and give yourself enough time to gather all the requested documents.

REMEMBER

You are in control of who you hire, partner with, or consult with to be a part of your care team. If you find yourself in a position where medical malpractice, negligence, or harm is suspected and you are considering working with an attorney or legal professional, the same mindset applies. Take time to interview as many experts as you need and work with the ones that work well with you.

Seek Out Crisis Aid

Along your journey, you may encounter life events that turn your world upside down, like losing your home, unemployment, mental health crises, and more. When these things happen, you need to know what support is available to you immediately and where to find it.

WARNING

If you are experiencing thoughts to hurt yourself or others, or other immediate threats to your safety, you can contact emergency services like 911 in the United States and suicide prevention hotlines, like 988. Remember you can also utilize a hospital's emergency department or community crisis centers.

It's best to be proactive and understanding what resources are available to you through nonprofit organizations, government programs, health systems, and others that can help you if you need food, shelter, medical attention, or refuge.

Keep an updated list of organizations that provide the support, their phone numbers and other crucial information. You live in a home with other people, especially children, make sure that they know who to call and what to say to get help for each situation. You can keep these important numbers and resources in a central location in your home where everyone can access them.

Work with Medical Bill Advocates and Finance Professionals

You already know that healthcare is expensive but what do you do when the bills start piling up, you have questions about the validity of your charges, or you need options for consolidating your debt? Working with a financial counselor or a medical bill advocate can help you strategize, understand the options available to you, and take some of the financial burden off.

The good news is that there are numerous resources and strategies available to help you address financial debt and stress in a way that is workable. The downside is that the average person probably doesn't know all of them. This is where a financial counselor or medical bill advocate can be very helpful. These professionals help identify errors in bills, facilitate the insurance claim filing process, negotiate lower bills, help you identify and apply for financial assistance programs, and much more. These powerhouse resources can help take the navigation burden off you while you focus on their wellness, health, and recovery.

Reach Out to Nonprofit Organizations

Some nonprofit organizations and community resources may have knowledge of programs and resources that can also offer support for free or at a reduced cost. Your state may also have a consumer assistance program, or CAP, that may be able to help you with some of your healthcare and insurance woes.

FIND ONLINE

For more information about CAPs, visit www.cms.gov/CCIIO/Resources/Consumer-Assistance-Grants.

Your health system may also have financial counselors or patient advocates that can help you free of charge within the parameters of their employment. For example, answering questions about a bill generated by the hospital. However, if you are dealing with challenges like considering bankruptcy due to overwhelming medical bills, disputing insurance claims, and so on, consider starting a conversation with a medical billing advocate or a local nonprofit.

Hire a Professional Interpreter

If you or a loved one has language barriers that prevent them from managing their own healthcare, this may be one professional that you can't live without.

Work with Financial Counselors and Advisors

Even with insurance, many patients still have financial obligations related to medical care. These financial obligations include co-payments, deductibles, co-insurance, and more. You can't predict when an accident happens or you will be diagnosed with a serious illness. However, financial advisors can advise you on how to best prepare to budget for your current and future health spending needs. Healthcare is not getting cheaper, so having a proactive plan to manage your money could potentially keep your expenses down. Financial advisors can be much more affordable and attainable than you think.

Gone are the days where the ultra-wealthy have a monopoly on the ability to afford professional services to make sure that they are saving, investing, and budgeting their money well. Take your time to find the right advisor for your needs, budget, and goals.

Financial advisors specialize in multiple types of money management — everything from estate planning to investing, so make a list of specific characteristics about your journey or need that you want advice on. For example:

- Are you turning 65 and wanting to budget for out-of-pocket medical expenses in the next couple of years?
- Have you been diagnosed with a serious illness and need help forecasting ways to handle the cost of serious illness care?

Write out your goals and the timeline in which you hope to achieve them. Evaluate your planner's credentials and look for additional financial planning related certifications like the Certified Financial Planner certification, as well as if they are *fiduciary*, meaning that they have made a commitment to act in the client's best interest, just to name a few.

Once you've narrowed down your list, start having conversations. Consider their communication styles, scope of work, and other business-related details for potential matches.

By planning for the cost of long-term care, yearly co-pays, or even medication expenses, you gain a level of control over your money. You can work with a specialized individual to provide a level of stability and foster a sense of resilience in preparedness for unexpected expenses.

Use Reputable Websites

Researching your situation on the web is never a bad idea, with the important caveat that you need to be sure that the sites you visit are reputable, honest, unbiased, and overall reliable. To begin, the Mayo clinic's site (`www.mayoclinic.org`) and WebMD (`www.webmd.com`) are good places to gather information about healthcare concerns, diagnoses, and more. Government-sponsored sites, such as MedlinePlus and `HealthCare.gov`, are also reliable.

WARNING

It bears repeating — don't believe just anything you read out there on the Internet. Anyone can post anything — which means the onus is on you to ensure you're getting truthful information. By using the sites mentioned here, you'll be in good stead.

For more advice on using the Internet, check out Chapter 8.

Work with a Private Patient Advocate

Nearly every healthcare professional in the industry can support and advocate for a patient within the confines of their role. Doctors, nurses, allied health professionals, and more do it all the time.

Even people outside of the traditional healthcare system, such as neighbors, families and friends, can advocate for another person.

But did you know that there is a whole *specialized* profession dedicated to helping patients manage the logistics of their healthcare, including everything from helping them improve relationships with their healthcare team, finding them the best ways to pay for their healthcare, and even coming with them to their doctors' appointments? These rockstars are called *private patient advocates.*

They can have a myriad of backstories that led them to do the work that they do. Some were patients themselves who had to learn how to navigate the healthcare system and survive; some were caregivers and support partners to loved ones and friends who were patients; some are practicing or retired nurses — the list goes on!

Backstories aside, private patient advocates are contracted to work for a patient and their family to provide them with a level of navigational and advocacy support that is individually tailored to that patient. They don't treat patients clinically, they don't recommend treatment plans, and they don't make decisions for you. However, they come alongside you and help you strategically navigate the healthcare system as a third party that is external to the emotion and exhaustion that patients and their families often feel.

REMEMBER

Private or independent patient advocates don't work for a hospital system or insurance company. Many of them have their own practices or firms where they work with patients as clients. It's very common for private patient advocates to be paid directly by their client and not take health insurance to cover their services, as working with the patient as a client directly allows the patient to be able to call all of the shots without conflicts.

If you feel like you're banging your head against the wall trying to get your care team to listen to you, you're overwhelmed with all the appointments you have to attend, you worry about if you're receiving the best care, or if you just want to experience the sheer bliss of having someone else help you coordinate your care and navigate the healthcare system, it's time to hire a patient advocate.

Where do you find patient advocates? There are directories online, such as Greater National Advocates, that list private, professional advocates. To be listed on these directories, some platforms require that advocates complete a background check, show proof of their relevant certifications (that also require background clearance), have professional liability insurance (like error and omission coverage), and more to make sure that the advocates you are screening are reputable.

REMEMBER

Never completely leave it up to a directory or a website to validate the integrity of any professional that you hire. It's your responsibility to do your own homework and ask the potential advocates questions to make sure they're a good fit for you.

Get Counseling or Therapy

Although they cannot address or treat your *medical* issues, counseling and therapy services can help you manage and deal with the mental aspects of long-term health conditions and provide you with ways to handle your maladies in a resilient and functional way.

Usually led by licensed mental health experts, therapy sessions can go a long way in giving you the "serenity to accept the things you cannot change, the courage to change the things you can, and the wisdom to know the difference," as the old saying goes.

IN THIS CHAPTER

» Starting a local garden

» Volunteering at health clinics

» Helping your community combat food waste

» Collaborating with your community to reduce preventable illnesses

Chapter 20
Ten Ways to Advocate for Health and Wellness in Your Community

By now you know the importance of advocating for your health and the impact that partnership and shared mission between you and your clinical team makes on the quality of healthcare you receive and your experience with the healthcare system. But how do you make a conscious effort to make your community healthier altogether and potentially prevent diseases? Advocating for health and wellness in your community is important because the environment that you live in has a direct impact on the health outcomes you experience.

This chapter contains actionable ways to foster community wellness and empower other community members to actively participate in health initiatives. This can ultimately make the difference between a healthy, happy community, and an unhappy, unhealthy one.

Start a Community Garden

Community gardens are gifts that keep on giving. In the shared space, members of the community have the opportunity to grow their own fruits and vegetables, benefit from physical activity of tending to the garden, as well as promote healthy eating. Not only do community gardens enhance the local wellness of a community by improving access to fresh produce, but they are also fun (see Figure 20-1)! To start a garden, you need:

- A great plot of land in an accessible, conducive location to allow plants to thrive
- A group of volunteers
- Educational initiatives to support concepts like sustainable composting or seasonal planning
- An equitable and sustainable system to share the harvest of the community garden with other community members in need.

A community garden can significantly impact your community's ability to be well and combat preventable chronic illnesses. One big reason that some people have trouble eating more fruits and vegetables is the availability and affordability of fresh produce.

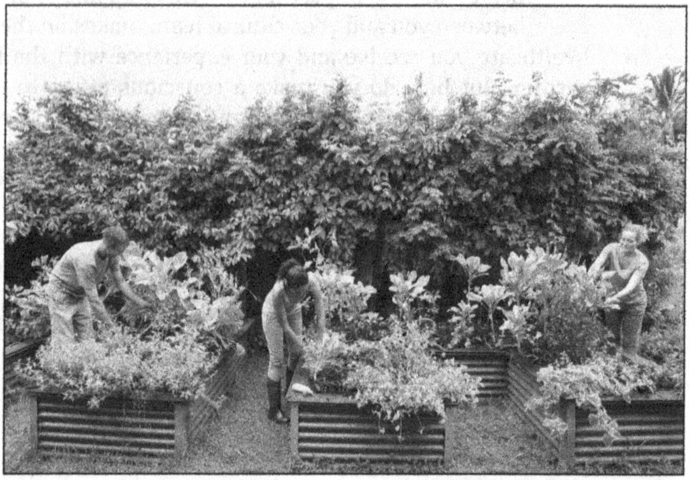

Gift Culture Media/KOTO/Adobe Stock Photos

FIGURE 20-1: Community gardens are a great way to provide healthy food while making connections with others.

TIP

If your community already has a garden, reach out to the initiative's leadership and ask how you can get involved. Asking questions about the current work, opportunities for improvement, and how you can help allows you to get involved in a impactful way and further the mission.

Get Involved with Local Fitness Classes

Keeping up a healthy level of physical activity and moving your body improves your mood and health, and even provide psychological benefits. Unfortunately, the ability to consistently work out and adhere to a fitness routine is not always easy, especially if you have limited income to pay for gym memberships, live in a city that doesn't have safe walking or running paths, or if you don't know where to start.

If you like physical activity, or maybe played sports at a point in your life, and you want to encourage physical activity among the residents of your community, consider working with or starting programs that offer free or inexpensive fitness classes to your community. Talk to your local community recreation centers about how you can get involved.

REMEMBER

You don't have to reinvent the wheel. Chances are there are programs out there that may have lost momentum in the recent months or years. Look into current offerings before you start your own. Use social media and other advertising to get the word out. Start with classes and fitness challenges that are fun to get people's attention. Consider asking local fitness instructors to join you to make professional guidance more accessible to a larger audience.

Work with Local Government Officials

Did you know that local government officials have more immediate impact to the health and wellness of a community compared to national or federal government officials? Being a well-informed community member and voter on all levels of government, makes you well equipped to understand the priorities of your government officials and hold them accountable for the health of your community.

Work with local authorities and government officials to implement policies and initiatives that prioritize public health and wellness in your community. You can advocate for issues such as safer parks and playgrounds, better access to healthy food, more walkable neighborhoods, and adding bike lanes, green spaces, and improving air quality.

REMEMBER

Government officials are busy people, so make sure that when you do present your concerns, your argument is well organized, succinct, and actionable. You want to come off as someone who can bring evidence-based data to support an issue and who clearly outlines specific initiatives and goals for improvement.

Many times, people remember the story you tell them more easily than the data you present. Give them a story to recount when it's time to vote on a particular bill, but substantiate your claims with data that makes sense. You must be able to speak their language, which could include statistics on health disparities in your community, the benefit of more walkable neighborhoods, lack of access to healthy food, and more.

TIP

Remember that your officials are people too and are passionate about different things. Make sure to do your homework on them before getting involved. Look for the overlap in your interests with theirs, the priorities of their office, and what policies or bills they support. If you get into the practice of being informed about the stance of your local government, you will be best equipped to vote for individuals who prioritize what you think is important and don't just talk the talk, but walk the walk.

Volunteer at Health Clinics and Initiatives

Many community members use health clinics to receive basic and primary care support for their health needs, especially if they are members of underserved populations or have limited financial resources.

Health clinics and many community-led health initiatives do great work with very few resources. They are essential to promoting community health and wellness and to ensure that people with chronic diseases can manage their care, improve access to wellness screenings, and provide essential health education. Volunteers may have the opportunity to help with administrative front-desk duties and patient intake to hands-on roles like patient transport and rooming. These organizations are usually ecstatic to welcome volunteers.

Keep a lookout for immunization drives, health fairs, and community health education opportunities. You can play an active role in the improvement of public health and community wellness in your neighborhood.

TIP

Do you have professional training as a nurse, a nursing or medical assistant, business manager, or something else related? Communicate that to the health clinic and initiative leadership. Volunteer opportunities may turn into permanent career opportunities as you build the relationship!

Organize a Community Clean-Up Event

Does the curb appeal of your community need a facelift? Consider organizing a community cleanup! Grab a group of volunteers and put together an event that gets members of the community outside, engaging in a little physical activity, and cleaning up the neighborhood. Excess amounts of trash pollution can have adverse effects on your community and subject your neighborhood to pests, like cockroaches and rats, transmitted diseases, water supply contamination, and more.

Not only does a community clean upkeep your neighborhood looking well-loved and healthy, it gives community members a sense of pride in the space they call home.

Support Local Schools to Encourage Healthy Practices

Healthy habits start at home — and at school. Healthier schools create healthier communities. Get involved with your local schools and look for opportunities to volunteer on committees or task forces that are committed to making the schools and students healthier. No change is too small! Whether you are picking a healthier snack alternative to send with your kids to soccer practice or working with your school district to advocate for and create health and wellness education initiatives, you're making a difference!

TIP

Don't know where to start? Reach out to local schools and ask about their healthy school initiatives. You can be connected with stakeholders who support everything from healthier cafeteria food options and mental health initiatives to physical activity initiatives and policy task forces.

Combat Food Waste in Your Home and Community

You probably heard it as a kid (or even told your own kids at the dinner table) to make sure you don't waste food and eat everything on your plate. Although the sentiment may be well-meaning in theory, there may be more effective ways to reduce food waste, within your home and within your community.

Addressing food waste from a community perspective fosters access to nutritional foods, healthy eating habits, and sustainability. Work with local programs and organizations to create educational programming that is focused on waste-limiting, strategic meal planning, cleaver tricks to store food and increase its longevity, or tasty recipes to make with leftovers from last night's dinner.

If you have a food bank in your community, ask them how you can get involved organizing or supporting their food drives. It's not uncommon for grocery stores to build initiatives that combat food-insecurity into their community impact and development plans. They may donate their surplus food to food banks and shelters.

Every year, tons of perfectly usable food goes to waste, which places stress on the physical environment as well as on community members who could have benefited from those goods. Whether you get a group of your neighbors to start composting or contribute to educational initiatives, every step toward preventing food waste contributes to a healthier community.

Advocate for More Accessible Communities

Accessibility is a crucial part of health and wellness because it has a direct impact on the lives of individuals who live, work, and play in the community that have disabilities, chronic conditions, or are older. City and urban planners, government agencies, businesses, and others have a civic responsibility to prioritize accessibility in the planning and creation of parks, public transportation systems, and businesses. However, many communities leave much to be desired in the conversation of accessibility. Accessibility affects people's options as to where they can live, work, shop, and recreate.

REMEMBER

The Americans with Disabilities Act (ADA) presents requirements and guidelines that hold businesses accountable to prioritize accessibility in public spaces. Business that do not prioritize accessibility not only miss out on a larger customer base, but can also be subjected to financial penalties and legal trouble.

Start a Walking Group

Looking to get active in a low-impact, cost-effective way? Chances are other members of your community are too! Start a walking group to foster a sense of community engagement and gain accountability to stay active and improve your health. If you have a group of interested people in mind, pick a meeting location and get to it. If you're looking for a group to join you, try advertising on a community center bulletin board or posting on social media. Before long, you will have a group of walkers who are committed to going on a self-paced walk a few times a month.

TIP

Want to keep your walks interesting? Consider assigning a theme to your walks that symbolize something fun, like a holiday party themed walk, scavenger hunts, or a bring-your-dog-to-the-walk day. Give away fitness-themed prizes for best walking shoes, most creative outfit, or friendliest pooch to keep things interesting. It might sound corny but some of the best memories are made around a cheesy themed event!

Prioritize Shopping Locally

Shopping locally and supporting small businesses positively impacts a community economically and socially. Local farmer's markets and vendors provide community members with access to fresh produce and other healthy foods that might not otherwise be available in the community without outsourcing them.

When you shop locally and encourage your friends and families to do the same, you not only support local businesses, which can encourage healthy consumer habits and provide healthy food choices, you also interact with members of your community and create connections that can support a sense of belonging, positively impacting the mental health of everyone involved.

IN THIS CHAPTER

» Blogging about your health journey

» Picking the best platforms for your storytelling style

» Making your experiences resonate with other people

Chapter 21
Ten Ways to Share Your Health Journey with Others

One of the fascinating things about healthcare journeys is that they are inherently unique, and no matter how similar your journey may be to another person's, they remain one-of-a-kind, just like the people who walk them. As you venture through the healthcare system, receiving a diagnosis, reaching treatment milestones, and building connections with clinical care teams, you cultivate a story that is just your own — transformative and empowering.

Maybe people have told you that others would benefit from hearing your story, or you have come to that conclusion on your own and are feeling overwhelmed with finding the best way to share it. Communicating your story in a way that is unique to you and empowers you to command the narrative not only helps the listener (or viewer) connect with you through the provision of comfort and guidance but can also help you blossom and showcase your best self as you confidently process your journey.

You've made the journey and gathered the courage to share (or you're still considering it), so it's time to explore a few meaningful and creative ways to tell your story in a way that might inspire others.

Start a Blog

Yes, blogging is still cool, and it can be a great way to journal your experiences. If you like to journal or are most comfortable with written testimonies, starting a blog might be a great option. There are many content styles you can adopt to communicate in your little corner of the Internet, with everything ranging from *listicles* (like this chapter listing ten ways to share your health journey with others) to videos, or even product reviews of your specially curated survival essentials.

TIP

Select a platform that helps you quickly post the content you want to share. Blogger or WordPress may work for you if you like a true-to-blog experience, while YouTube may be the best platform for video blogs (vlogs). A mixture of both can also work!

Share Your Story in Online Communities

One of the main reasons that patients and their support teams seek out online communities is because they are looking for a safe space where people can speak openly about their experiences and provide support, comfort, and guidance as they navigate the terrain of a shared illness or condition. People want to hear from other patients who understand their situation. Research online, disease-specific communities to contribute to. These groups can be interactive, collaborative, and informative — virtual "water coolers" for sharing insight, asking questions, and sharing perspectives.

WARNING

Patient online communities have evolved over the years, from everything from email listservs and online discussion boards to patient communities on Facebook and Reddit, and even their own dedicated platforms. Many platforms advertise that they are specifically geared toward providing patients with opportunities to build community with others from specific disease groups. While this advancement is an excellent step in the right direction, it is crucial to be mindful of the communication you share and to practice decorum as you interact with other members.

Don't give out personal information that you wouldn't want other people to share without your permission. Be mindful that everyone is at a different stage in their health journey, so be kind and non-judgmental in your communication.

Record Your Journey and Create a Channel Online

Video content can be a very impactful medium for sharing stories in a personal and familiar manner. Many content creators record vlogs, video shorts or reels, and other video content that allows their followers to glimpse into their daily lives. You can start by recording videos on your phone and acting like you're talking to a friend. You can talk about your experiences, your thoughts (or even fears) about the current situation you're navigating, or even give advice and respond to questions or comments some viewers may leave for you as you build your following and post on a social platform, like Instagram or YouTube. This is a great option for those who like to be in front of the camera.

Whether you're about to get ready for a doctor's appointment or preparing to wind-down for the night, you can record a quick video check-in to keep your followers updated. Your daily life on your wellness journey is more interesting and valuable than you might think, especially for people on a similar path.

TIP

You don't have to record every aspect of your journey to be relatable. Make a content posting plan each month. For example, if you know you meet with your clinician every third Tuesday, you can plan to record something related to your health journey on those days. Have fun with the process. There's no rule book, so make the expression your own.

Start a Podcast

Podcasts allow you to share your story in "episodes" through spoken words. Like audiobook lovers, people who enjoy listening to content gravitate toward this form of self-expression. You can record episodes on various topics about your journey or condition(s) to tell your story, give advice, offer opinions, and more. As you grow along your podcast journey, you can invite guests you admire or who share similar experiences with you to dialogue with you. You can take it a step further and ask your audience to send in questions for you to answer on the next episode.

TIP

Want to sound professional even though you just started your podcast? Do research online about the best equipment to invest in to give your audience a good listening experience. Many resources include a range of options to invest in, from beginner, cost-efficient equipment to advanced investment pieces.

Write a Book

Have you ever shared you story with someone, and they responded, "I think you should write a book!"? They may be on to something! In a book, you can effectively convey the depth of your journey without getting in front of a camera or behind a microphone. You can hire professionals to help you get your manuscript published, or you can self-publish your book on platforms like Amazon Kindle. Some authors choose to release their book for free as an e-book. You have many options for getting your book out there, but the first thing is to write it.

Become a Freelance Writer

Many popular health websites, magazines, and forums compensate freelance writers for sharing their stories and insights on a specific topic. If you like sharing your story through the written word, this option may be particularly attractive to you. Think about the topics you can write about while providing helpful insights. Once you've identified those things, research health blogs or newsletters that align with your content in substance and style.

Participate in Advocacy Campaigns

Patient self-advocacy is a part of the patient advocacy movement. The more you know about the healthcare system, the better your clinical outcomes and experience with the healthcare system can be. But how do you work to change the healthcare delivery system so that you and other patients don't have to fight as hard? You can get involved with advocacy campaigns!

Through these channels, you can share your story with key changemakers, like elected officials, and contribute to the mission of enhancing the visibility of your condition or stumbling blocks in your journey while advocating for change. Many disease-specific organizations (such as the American Cancer Society or the Alzheimer's Association) have campaigns related to specific conditions that allow people to share their stories with policymakers and contribute to awareness events.

Speak at Events or on Webinars

Got the gift of gab? Speaking engagements allow you to share your story in person, on a live stream, or webinar and connect directly to your audience. You can reach out to organizations in your community or organizations that you admire to get information about opportunities to provide your patient perspective. There are a variety of speaking formats available outside of keynote speakers. For example, you could speak on a panel with other patients.

TIP

Speaking in real time to an audience can be overwhelming, especially if you suffer from anxiety or stage fright. It's important to remember that the people are there to hear *your* story. You don't have to pretend to be someone or something that you're not to convey your story in an impactful way.

Communicate Through Art and Photography

Not only is art a therapeutic, powerful, and individualized way to express your experience and feelings, it can also be a impactful medium to communicate to other people. If you like to draw, paint, take pictures, create sculptures, write music, or something else, consider using your experiences as the subject of some of your art. Your healthcare journey is as private as you'd like it to be, so there's no harm in creating artistic pieces to symbolize your journey and keeping them for yourself or those close to you. If you feel inclined to share your art with the world, consider partnering with galleries in your community or sharing your art online. Maybe you found an artistic solution to a challenge you experienced on your healthcare journey and want to make it available to other patients. If so, consider selling it on websites geared toward one-of-a-kind pieces or handcrafted art, such as Esty.

Contribute to Clinical Research

Some patients' journeys through the healthcare system are more complicated because there isn't enough scientific research or information about their condition. To make matters worse, the research that clinicians and pharmaceutical companies do have about certain conditions might not fully represent all the patient populations that live with them — they don't have enough information from patients of different ethnicities, socioeconomic statuses, genders, ages, and so on. Ask your clinical care team about research studies that apply to your condition.

TIP

If there aren't any research studies available through your health system, consider searching for trials on `ClinicalTrials.gov`, which is sponsored by the National Institutes of Health (NIH).

If you are interested in research, or have a background in science, and you don't see a study on your condition that aims to answer the questions you have, ask your clinician to connect you with researchers at your institution or a university who may be interested in designing a study with your questions in mind. You may have the opportunity to contribute to the field of research and publish research findings. You may also be offered the chance to present at conferences.

Managing multiple or complex health conditions can make it difficult to work a full-time (or even part-time) job and have a consistent income, which leads to financial stress for many patients. However, sharing your story in these ways may present opportunities for compensation. This financial support can alleviate some of the stress and uncertainty, allowing you to focus more on your health and well-being.

IN THIS CHAPTER

- » Celebrating your healthcare wins by throwing a party
- » Sending out gratitude to those who helped you
- » Donating to a worthy cause
- » Creating a victory playlist

Chapter 22 Ten Ways to Celebrate Your Healthcare Wins and Milestones

Navigating the healthcare system is hard and advocating for yourself along the way can feel even harder. That's why, when you meet a significant milestone in your journey, you need to celebrate it! Recognizing your successes and progress not only makes you feel good, but it also reinforces the positive behaviors that helped you achieve them. You've done hard work and come out on top! It's time to grab a party favor and learn some fun ways to celebrate your accomplishments. Celebrating can motivate you to keep advocating for your health.

Commemorate Your Wins

Take pictures of the day and scrapbook them in an album dedicated to your healthcare journey or post them on social media. However you choose to share your wins and milestones, make an intentional effort to capture the moment when you finish your last chemotherapy treatment, organize all your medications for the month, or stand up for yourself during an appointment when you're not being heard (just to name a few).

TIP

Not a big fan of social media? Send the picture you snapped to a few close friends or family members in a group chat. Fine with a party of one? Make a dedicated photo album in your phone's photo gallery of your wins and save them for yourself!

Throw a Party!

What better way to celebrate your accomplishments than to throw a party! Grab your family, friends, and supporters, a couple of party favors, a great playlist, and make the day one to remember. Theme your party around one of your victories and ask your guests to join in.

REMEMBER

It's not the size of the guest list that matters — it's the quality! Don't feel like you have to roll out a Met Gala-sized guest list to have a good time. A party with 5 people can be just as fun as a party with 50 people (it's also way less clean up).

Eat Your Favorite Meal

Cook (or order) your favorite meal to celebrate your victory! Ask your family and friends to pitch in with the prep or join you in a nice meal at your favorite restaurant (or on your couch) to make the event even more special. Bonus points to you if you enjoy a healthier version of your favorite meal!

Send Your Care Team a Celebratory Thank You

Write and send thank-you notes to members of your clinical support team, front-desk staff, and support partners thanking them for their help in achieving your goals. People who have a vested interest in you feeling and living better, like your care team, love to hear that you're making progress. Your wins can brighten their day, so share that great feeling!

Treat Yourself to Some Rest and Relaxation

You've earned it — now it's time to rest. Plan a trip to a spa, go for a hike, get a massage, schedule a day off work to binge watch your favorite TV show, or do something else that you enjoy. Whether you opt for an elaborate getaway or simply get a pedicure, making an intentional effort to reward yourself reinforces your winning behaviors with wellness and rest.

Buy Yourself Something Special

Buy a memento or special treat that symbolizes your victory, such as a piece of jewelry, a latte, or something else that you would otherwise pass on but would like to have. It doesn't have to be expensive but should make your day feel a bit more special (because it is).

Donate to a Cause You Care About

Sometimes the best gift is the one you give to someone else. Make a donation to an organization whose mission you care about or one that helped you get through a hard time. Consider donating to a nonprofit organization that fights to find a cure for your condition or supports other people living with it.

Dress Up for the Occasion

You know that outfit in the back of your closet that you've been looking for an excuse to wear? You just found it! Get dressed up and go someplace special, walk in the park, or just sit in the living room. Dressing up can make you feel good about how you look and can solidify the message that what you've achieved is a big deal and is worth celebrating.

Make Your Space Festive

Decorate your environment with balloons, streamers, or other decorations that make you happy. Display some fresh flowers and other things that you like in your home, office, or wherever you find yourself. Anything that reminds you to celebrate your significant achievements is fair game.

Create a Victory Playlist

Make a playlist dedicated to your victory! Add songs that empower you, make you laugh, or inspire you, and play them when you meet a goal.

TIP

You can send your family and friends a link to contribute to the playlist. Build your playlist and play it at your next gathering — or jam out by yourself at home!

IN THIS APPENDIX

» Using digital voice recorders to track your health information

» Arranging your appointments with a calendar app

» Accessing your patient portal

» Trying wearable technology

Appendix A
Using Technology to Stay Organized

One of the most significant upsides of technology is that it can simplify your life and streamline your current processes. The more you can automate or use technology to "think" about the small stuff, such as keeping your calendar and organizing multiple doctor's appointments, the more time you have to focus on the bigger, more important things, like relationship building and self-care.

Technology changes daily, so new tools and features are constantly developed to help you stay organized. Don't be afraid to experiment and find what works best for you.

Using Digital Voice Recorders for Appointments

Chances are, if you are like most patients, you've sat through one (or more) doctor's appointments trying to catch all the critical details that your provider is telling you while scribbling notes on the back of an envelope or piece of paper you found at the bottom of your tote bag. Been there?

A voice recorder is one of the simplest and most effective ways to capture important information. Most smartphones have a voice memo app installed, where you press the big button and begin recording. If you don't have a smartphone, you can buy a physical voice recorder or another dictation device (see Figure A-1). You can also use a voice recorder to leave messages to yourself about your care. If you are a visual person who likes to read notes, you can even convert your audio recordings into transcripts using a transcription app.

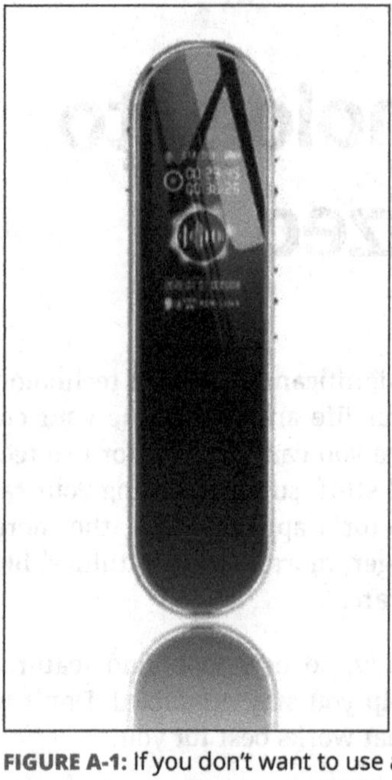

FIGURE A-1: If you don't want to use an app on a smartphone, you can buy a simple voice recorder like the XENO here to record all your conversations with your care team.

(c) Zetronix Corp.

TIP

Before your next appointment, make a list of any questions have and try to stick to it as best you can to ensure that your recording is focused and doesn't get bogged down with irrelevant information.

REMEMBER

Ask for your doctor or provider's permission to record the conversation. Even if you have the right to record the conversation without letting your provider know, it's better to be upfront about your intention to record the conversation. That way, your provider doesn't feel like you are trying to catch them doing or saying something wrong, potentially leading to a guarded and strained relationship.

Organizing Your Appointments with a Calendar App

Believe it or not, people used to have to manage their appointments by hand on a paper calendar (or datebook if you want a real throwback). Some people prefer to keep this same method because it works for them, and there are different strokes for different folks. The good news is that if you find writing appointments, circling important dates in various colors, and crossing out canceled appointments tedious and inefficient, technology allows you to manage your calendar electronically.

Many calendar apps integrate seamlessly with other productivity tools you use daily — such as email, task managers, or project management software — to create a more cohesive and integrated experience that keeps you from switching between platforms. You can use calendar apps to add events, like upcoming doctor appointments, to your calendars and even set reminders. You can also change the frequency and duration of the reminder to best suit your needs. Consider playing around with the options until you find ones that fit you best.

Calendar apps are easy to customize and even provide options to color-code specific events. It's now super easy to reschedule or cancel an appointment using these apps. Another plus is that calendar apps can synchronize to all your devices, including your phone and computer, making it very easy to navigate your schedule as it changes whenever and wherever you are.

TIP

If you wear multiple hats and have many responsibilities, like many patients do, or maybe you are managing your healthcare as well as the healthcare of a loved one, it might be a good idea to electronically share each other's calendar app. This way, if you're trying to coordinate schedules with other family members or friends, you can do so more easily.

Building a Health Accountability Plan with a Digital Task Manager

Managing your healthcare can feel like a project, literally. So why not manage it like one? There are parts of the "project" owned by you as the patient, such as calling to schedule an appointment to meet with your specialist, and parts owned by your clinician, such as signing prior authorization paperwork. Task management apps — like Asana and Trello — offer a free trial of premium features before you have to pay to upgrade to the premium version. The free version works well enough if you're using the application to keep yourself organized.

Once you've found an application you like, you can organize your health-related tasks into categories like medication schedules, to-do lists, follow-ups, and appointments. In these categories, you can select due dates for each task. You can log an appointment as a milestone and make the due date the day of the appointment. You can also set a due date for refilling a medication. Setting deadlines for tasks you must complete can help you stay organized and manage your time.

TIP

Make time regularly — every week or monthly — to review your plan. Start playing around with the application, ensuring your tasks are updated when you create and complete something, and reassess your needs along your health journey.

WARNING

Not all digital task managers are HIPAA compliant. Refrain from adding personal data to these applications, including your birth date, Social Security number, or other info that can be harmful if it were accessed by someone else.

Using the Patient Portal

Patient portals, like MyChart, are the command central for patients managing multiple aspects of their healthcare and, if used correctly, can enhance your experience.

Patient portals can streamline many aspects of your healthcare experience. They make it easy to access important information and services right from the comfort of your computer or phone. If you're not familiar with the patient portal that your hospital system uses, make it a point to find out. Once you have gained access to the portal, familiarize yourself with your profile on the portal. Figure A-2 shows an example the MyChart dashboard.

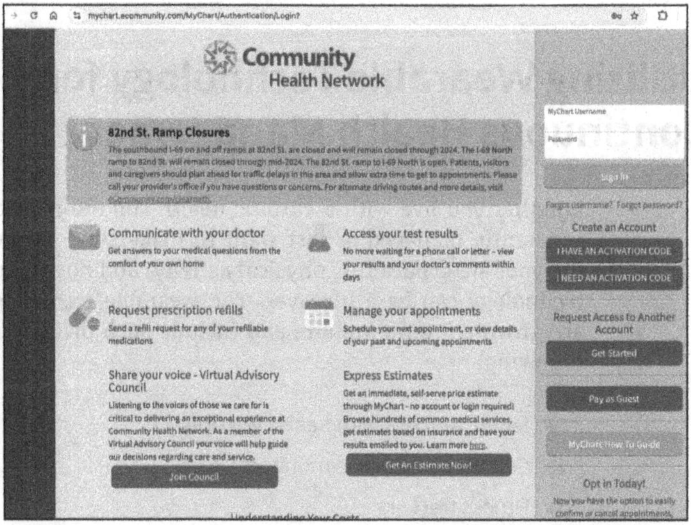

FIGURE A-2: Your patient portal contains information about your visits, lab results, upcoming tests, messages from your care team, and more.

TIP

Double-check the information on your portal. Be sure that your name is spelled correctly, your contact information is accurate, and your insurance information is up to date. From this portal, you can view any after-visit notes from your healthcare providers as well as your test results as they come in. You can also review and access information like your current medications, allergies, and more. By keeping this information up to date, you minimize the chance of an error or a miscommunication.

You can also send your care team a message or request an appointment from most portals. You can review available appointment times and fill out pre-appointment questionnaires, which will make the moments leading up to your appointment much more peaceful. Some patient portals allow you to set reminders about medication refills and appointments. Some even allow you to request prescription refills right through the portal.

By using your patient portal, you can be proactive about your healthcare information and the management of your care.

TIP

Some health systems offer instructions for using their patient portals. Ask your doctor's office to connect you with the appropriate departments or to send you some resources on how to download, log in, and navigate your patient portal.

Utilizing Wearable Technology for Continuous Health Management

Whether you live with a chronic health condition that has to be constantly managed or just want to make sure you are managing your sleep patterns, physical activity, and nutrition, wearable technology can be a lifesaver. The wearable technology options are growing by the minute and include such diverse uses as the following:

- Smart watches with health features
- Continuous glucose monitors
- Fitness trackers
- Remotely programmed hearing aids
- Heart rate trackers
- Mobile ECG devices
- Fertility trackers

They collect important metrics about your health like your sleep patterns, heart rate, physical activity, and more. Having access to large amounts of real-time data can empower you and your healthcare team to make important decisions about your health and wellness.

As data is collected, many platforms allow you to view your stats, giving you the opportunity to review your personalized data. You can then start or continue conversations with your care team about ways to stay healthy, your concerns, preventative measures, and other insights.

Talk to your clinical team about what kind of data you should collect and monitor. Once you have a good idea of the information you want to gather and continuously monitor, research which wearable devices, like smart watches, fitness trackers, and even smartphone apps, collect and present that data in ways that will be helpful and empowering to you. You can opt for the newest technology out there or simply use your smartphone.

TIP

If you have a solid idea of what information you're looking to review, you don't always have to splurge on the latest and greatest technology. Some tried-and-true devices and apps you already use might do the trick.

TIP

Some insurance plans and employee wellness initiatives provide incentives for meeting specific health metrics. Utilizing wearable technology could provide value in other parts of your coverage. You never know — you might get credited for purchasing these devices and therefore offset your out-of-pocket costs.

Make sure that you make decisions about your health with your personal care team; this ensures that your interpretation of the results is accurate.

IN THIS APPENDIX

» Finding a supportive online community

» Safely engaging with support communities

» Creating your own online support system

» Taking a relationship offline

Appendix B
Accessing Online Support Communities

Digital communities are everywhere. Whether you are a beauty influencer, social activist, or a sports fan there is a digital community on almost every social media platform to connect people who share the same beliefs, belong to the same groups, identify with the same values with each other so that they can connect share successes, tips of the trade, or even seek help from those who are similar to them.

Whether you are considering joining an existing community, wanting to know where to start, or considering creating your own space, understanding the dynamics, benefits, and additional considerations is crucial to your success.

In this appendix, you learn the importance of community, how to stay safe when interacting in online forms, ways to engage with others, and more.

Understanding Why Online Support Communities Matter

Digital spaces allow individuals to connect in person, regardless of geographic location, schedules, or other factors. People can come together with a shared identity or interest and provide a sense of belonging, identify opportunities to navigate challenges, and support others everywhere.

Communities can provide a level of support, camaraderie, and visibility to patients who may otherwise feel like they are all alone. Community, digital or not, can have significant positive impacts to a person's individual journey.

Support communities can provide patients, who may otherwise feel alone on a niche journey, empowerment and validation that their experiences are relevant and shared. It's like feeling like you belong to a team. Being a part of a community can improve your emotional well-being, provide you additional insights or ideas to address specific problems, and so much more.

Vetting an Online Community

What do you want out of an online community? Consider these factors:

- **Reflect on the identities that are the most prominent for you.** Maybe your role as a caregiver to an aging parent and a parent of small children are too prominent identities in your life. Both roles come with a multitude of responsibilities, and you may find it difficult to care for those around you, your parents and your children, while still doing the things you enjoy, and, placing a specific emphasis on your healthcare, manage your multiple health conditions as well.

  You might benefit from finding a community of patients who are also caregivers to their aging parents as well. Or you could consider joining a community of patients who are managing their health conditions and raising kids — or a mixture of the two.

- **Look for communities where people share similar roles and responsibilities.** The nuances of caring for someone else while caring for yourself presents additional considerations and potentially challenges that patients who don't have lifestyles that require them to focus on caretaking of many other people may not recognize or consciously create safe spaces to problem solve and make the journey a bit easier.
- **Note each group's mission, purpose of the group, communication style, as well as community tone and membership engagement.** Interact with spaces that matched what is important to you. It is important to you to use your experience as a patient to educate policymakers and lawmakers about issues that can affect the care people with the condition that you have, there are groups for that. If you are passionate about meeting up with people in a fun social way that share the same condition you do, there are groups for that.

  If you are looking for communities that help patients navigate pregnancy and the management of a specific condition, there may be groups for that as well! Interacting with social support communities should benefit you, in your ability to gather insights, support, and meet interesting people with different perspectives, as well as it should the community, by giving you a platform to interact and share your perspectives as well with other people.

TIP

You are a multifaceted human being who has several identities, which means that you may belong to a number of different patient support communities! Some communities will support the overlap of different identities you have, while other ones may just be tailored towards other people like you that just share a particular one.

Take time to research and explore different communities to find which ones stick for you. Here are some additional things to consider when looking for support communities.

Are privacy and security priorities?

Your healthcare journey is personal. Be careful how you share personal information on social platforms and make sure your community follows HIPAA compliance guidelines as well. Research how your data will be collected and utilized. Does the platform have alternative or financial interests in working with other organizations to persuade you to use the resources?

Can you participate anonymously?

Not every platform offers this option. However, having the option to participate anonymously may be a differentiating factor for you, so consider this issue when deciding on a platform..

How are inappropriate, harmful, or hurtful comments handled?

Many support forums, geared towards providing patience support communities or not, do have a code of conduct that users must abide by in order to participate on the platform.

For platforms that have made it a priority to ensure that users interact with each other in a respectful, constructive way, community guidelines and code of conduct policies are easy to spot and often required by the site for users to acknowledge their review and acceptance of that policy prior to moving into a portion of the space where they can interact with others.

Are your interactions with other community members positive?

Let's be real, there are so many parts of the healthcare journey that are hard, tear jerking, frustrating, and downright maddening.

Pay attention to how others respond to posts or messages like this. There isn't any kind of expectation for anyone to virtually rub anyone on the back and tell them everything will be okay just for the sake of saying it, but you should feel like the peer-to-peer interaction between members is overall supportive.

Does the platform have good reviews?

At the end of the day, it's your experience with a particular website, forum, or platform that holds the most weight in whether you feel it's appropriate to be a part of the community; however, looking at reviews of other users about the platform and what their experience was like may help you make your decision clearer.

It's common for users to talk about how easy it is to navigate a form or community, how accessible the platform is for those who are living with disabilities, things they found helpful, as well as opportunities for improvement. As with any feedback you receive from a third party, take it with a grain of salt and come to a conclusion about the topic on your own, but be open to reviewing other people's experiences as well if you would like to have a well-rounded set of data to analyze.

Does the platform prioritize ads over content?

Take a look at how much web page real estate is allocated to advertising. Is the platform trying to sell you something? Is it promoting the use of a brand-name drug? Does it feel gimmicky? Ultimately, you want to be a part of a community platform whose mission is to provide you a collaborative space to meet with patients on a similar journey as you, not to push a product or sell you on something.

Safely Engaging in Support Communities

Once you find a community, or communities, that provides a safe space to amplify the voices of patients who are navigating journeys similar to yours, it's important to understand how to not only be an act member of the community, but how to engage with other community members, interact in a positive way, and keep yourself and others safe.

Here are some tips for making the most of your experience in an online support community.

Be careful what you share online

You've probably already heard it before but the Internet is forever. Yes, there are protections you can take to protect your identity and your information online; however, nothing is ever foolproof. Approach posting anything on the Internet with the caveat of asking yourself "How would I feel if this information made it to people I didn't know?"

Your level of comfort is ultimately your best gage as to what information you want to share with the world and what should remain private, but some general pieces of information that you should keep to yourself are things like your social security number, your medical record number, your home address, and your bank account information keep to yourself.

Everyone is different and some people don't mind being very vocal about a bad experience they had with a provider or a medication they took and had a bad experience with, while others are more compatible being reserved.

A rule of thumb to abide by is to only consider posting things that you wouldn't mind being discussed in rooms where you are not present or conversations you wouldn't mind having outside the comfort of your home.

Be respectful of every member

You are fully entitled to your opinion and so are other people, even if it's different from yours. Being different from one another is what makes us unique and on a very personal self-advocacy journey, and on the plight to wellness, everyone has different priorities, once, needs, and goals that are specific to them and their situation. If you disagree with something that someone says, avoid responding in a way that can be perceived as a personal attack to someone else.

You can disagree with someone's judgment without calling them stupid or without insulting them.

If someone is uncomfortable sharing more information about an experience that they've had or doesn't want to engage as fully as some other members in various conversations, respect their boundaries and don't pressure anyone to have conversations or share information they're uncomfortable sharing.

Treating people the way that you would want to be treated it is a timeless adage that should be applied to every social interaction people have with each other. You can disagree without being disagreeable.

Make an intentional effort to stay on topic

Because certain online forums, like Reddit, have sub threads that are a dedicated place to talk about a subtopic of a topic, you could be a part of a community of patients who are managing attention-deficit/hyperactivity disorder or ADHD and participating in a conversation about behavioral changes. This wouldn't be the best part of the forum to talk about your experience finding the right medication because there's probably a dedicated space for that elsewhere.

One of the benefits of online support communities is that many conversations can be allocated to specific categories making it easy for members to find a topic that is relevant to them and participate in it without being subjected to tangents or the introduction of off-topic conversations. Just as you would like to benefit from organized focused discussions, give other people the opportunity by asking yourself if what you're posting is relevant to the place in where you're posting it.

Be mindful of the language you use in public spaces

It's helpful to read the room and assess what kind of tone in language is appropriate for that setting. Some people are not particularly bothered by profanity while others are sensitive to it.

Avoid being confrontational, using excessive profane language, or conducting yourself in a way that could be considered off putting or offensive to others.

Creating Your Own Support Community

Although there are thousands of support communities dedicated to different diseases, walks of life of patients managing them, geographic locations, and more, an online support community for the narrative or identity you have or your condition may not exist yet. This can occur for patients who are undiagnosed, or have a rare disease. Even though the support community may not exist yet doesn't mean that you have to wait around for someone to create one — you can consider creating one yourself! Consider these questions and tips as you get started creating a space for you, and other people like you, to connect.

Identify the typical community member

As you build your platform laser focus on who your community should be for initially. Is the community for people managing a particular health condition and working full-time? Is it for people with a specific rare disease? Is it for loved ones and caregivers of patients managing a specific condition?

The answer to these questions doesn't have to be completely exhaustive, but you do need to have a clear idea of where you need to start. It's not uncommon for people that create their own support community. Maybe you are a pastry chef with celiac disease and want to create an online community for other pastry chefs who are navigating their journey with celiac disease. Maybe you are an academic with an executive functioning disorder and want to create a community for other people in higher education who are managing similar conditions.

Whatever your niche group looks like be able to identify it and don't be scared to revisit and expand on it later to make it more inclusive. Make an intentional effort to define what the group is supposed to do. Is it an accountability group? A great space to meet and greet? Is it something different?

Answer these questions when creating your group:

1. Make it clear what community members would benefit from by being a part of the community. Ask yourself why someone should join your community. Are you offering peer support? Is there educational content and information being shared? Will you collaborate with healthcare professionals to create educational content? Spotlight the personal experiences of community members to foster a sense of community.

TIP

Think about the value of your group from the position of someone who's deciding if they want to join. Even if you've identified multiple perks to a members involvement in your group, ask yourself if that information is relayed clearly to community members.

WARNING

Be very careful about the providing medical advice in online support communities. Keep in mind that everyone's individual journey, disease presentation, and circumstances are different so the determination of what clinical interventions, therapies, or services that a patient and community members should endure should be made between them and their personal clinical care team.

Of course, there is nothing wrong with reading about someone else's experience with a clinical intervention or listening to their. Just because a medication work for you, doesn't mean that it will work for me and vice versa.

Websites and communities often have a disclaimer on their website indicating that they are not providing medical advice or treatment and that clinical decisions should be made with a licensed medical professional involved in that person's specific care.

2. Figure out where your community will live on the Internet and what platform will host it. Will your community be hosted on a website and function as a blog? Will you use an app to create a community? Will your group be a Reddit community, Facebook group, or something different? Will you create a community on an existing health community platform? Consider your options and weigh the pros and cons of each approach. Be sure to consider privacy, accessibility, and user friendliness as you decide where your platform will be.

3. Consider how you will get engagement and new members. Imagine you had a smoothie shop that made the best smoothies in town. Everyone who came into your shop and tried your smoothies raved about how great they were, but you weren't getting a lot of traffic Because you weren't making an intentional effort to let people know about how great your shop was. The same thing can happen with great support communities.

Consider how you'll get the word out about your community. Will you use social media, collaborate with patient advocacy organizations who already have an audience of patients looking for empowerment? Will you invest in search engine optimization or SEO to drive traffic to your website?

You don't have to have all the answers right now, but it helps to have an idea of how you will spread the word about the amazing support community you're building.

TIP

Get to know the leadership of similar online patient support groups and let them know about your platform and the community. As people get to know that your community, people that belong to one community may start to mention your community to others. There may be opportunities to cross collaborate, share insights on running the community, or just build a pleasant professional relationship.

TIP

As you build your community, make it clear to community members which actions, conversations, and behaviors are acceptable and which are not. If disputes arise, misinformation is shared or disrespectful behavior occurs, have a clear plan as to how you will address it per your community guidelines.

Taking Community Relationships Safely Offline

As you find communities of people who share common interests, common conditions, and even identities, you may build relationships that can transition from the digital space to a real life interaction. The people you connect with may live in your same city, attend your same religious institution, or go to your same school. If you are considering taking the opportunity to meet in person with a community member you've met through online support forums, you have to ensure that those in-person interactions are. Here are some tips to consider for safely taking community relationships offline.

1. **Have your first meeting in a neutral, public place.** Even if you feel like you've known the person you're meeting for a long time, or even if you have known them for a long time through the online community, it's always a good idea to arrange your first in-person meeting in a place that is neutral, public, and well populated. Avoid meeting in places like your home, and opt to meet at places like a casual restaurant, coffee shop or community event. It's important to make sure

that everyone feels comfortable with the meeting place. It's not cynical to prioritize your safety in meeting someone In person for the first time.

TIP

If the person or people you are meeting insists on meeting in a place that you're not comfortable with or that you feel is secluded, that may be a red flag. In a situation like this, reaffirm your preference to meet in someplace in public and if you continue to be uncomfortable with their persistence, you always have the option not to meet at all.

2. **Don't be afraid to set boundaries.** You don't have to do anything that you don't want to do. Make sure that everyone is on the same page. Just like in one line conversations, be mindful of how much personal information you share with your new connection. Relationships evolve over time and that there's nothing wrong with sharing more information about yourself as you get to know a person.
3. **Let someone you trust know where you will be before you meet anyone in person.** On many smart phones, you can simply share your location with a family or a friend when you are on your way to meet someone offline for the first time. Let them know where you will be meeting, what time you'll be meeting, who you will be meeting, and when you expect to be back.

TIP

Have you ever met someone and you got talking and time just flew by? Sometimes that happens and it's not a bad thing. Consider setting yourself a reminder to give that person a call or send them a text at the time you expected to be back if your meeting time is running longer than you anticipated. You could also ask your friend or loved one to give you a call at a certain time to check in with you to make sure everything is going well.

4. **Trust your gut when meeting someone in person.** If you feel like something is off, something is probably off. If, for any reason, you begin to feel uncomfortable or unsafe, you can politely cut the interaction short, cancel the meeting, or seek appropriate help.

WARNING

If you feel like you are in danger in any way should way, shape, or form, reach out to law enforcement or get the attention of someone else at the venue to get out of harm's way quickly and safely.

Index

C

D

E

F

G

H

I

J

K

L

M

N

O

P

Q

R

U

V

W

About the Author

Nichole Davis, DHA, MPH, BCPA, is a passionate patient-turned-patient advocate and innovative social impact entrepreneur committed to transforming the healthcare experience by helping patients understand and navigate the healthcare system.

After navigating the complexities of the healthcare system as a patient and as a professional patient advocate, she has dedicated her career to advocating for a more equitable system that places patients and their families at the center of their own care. She is the founder of Wayfinder Patient Advocates, a private patient advocacy practice dedicated to making healthcare simple for everyone by giving patients the tools they need to have a better healthcare experience.

Dr. Davis is a Board-Certified Patient Advocate (BCPA) who specializes in empowering patients while assisting them in navigating their healthcare with empathy. Her work has sparked vital conversations about patient experience and empowerment.

She's been recognized by Crain's Cleveland Business, *Modern Healthcare,* and *Forbes* as a leader and a change agent in the healthcare and public health industries.

To learn more about her work and upcoming projects, visit `www.wayfinderpatientadvocates.com`.

Dedication

This book is dedicated to all patients and caregivers who navigate the healthcare systems every day. You are stronger, more resilient, and more inspiring than you think.

To my family, mentors, and friends — thank you for your love, support and guidance. It means more to me than you know.

Acknowledgments

Thank you to the Wiley team, especially Jennifer Yee and Kezia Endsley, for their patience and faith in me as this book was brought to life. I could not have asked for a better team.

To my fellow patient advocates, thank you for continuing to give me hope in our mission and inspire me to continue to advocate for change. To the Wayfinder Patient Advocates community, your stories, insights, and determination have shaped this book, and I am deeply grateful for every conversation and every moment of shared experience. Thank you for reminding me daily why this work matters.

Lastly, thank you — readers — for trusting me to help make sense of the healthcare system.

Publisher's Acknowledgments

Acquisitions Editor: Jennifer Yee

Managing Editor: Murari Mukundan

Senior Project/Copy Editor: Kezia Endsley

Production Editor: Saikarthick Kumarasamy

Cover Image: © SDI Productions/ Getty Images